Life of bone

art meets science

Contributors

- Joni Brenner
- Elizabeth Burroughs
- Debbie Glencross
- Donald Johanson
- Gerhard Marx
- Karel Nel
- Kopano Ratele
- Lynne Slonimsky
- Himla Soodyall
- Bernhard Zipfel

Editors

Joni Brenner

Elizabeth Burroughs

Karel Nel

WITS UNIVERSITY PRESS

FRONT COVER AND TITLE PAGE (DETAIL): Border Cave 1 cranium of *Homo sapiens*, lateral left. Photograph by Dr Gerald Newlands, 1992, courtesy of Faculty of Health Sciences, University of the Witwatersrand.

Wits University Press
1 Jan Smuts Avenue
Johannesburg
South Africa
http://witspress.wits.ac.za

First published 2011

ISBN 978-1-86814-539-3

Edited by Vanessa Perlman
Proofread by Pat Botes
Design and layout by Karel Nel, Joni Brenner and Kevin Shenton
Printed and bound by Ultra Litho (Pty) Limited

Life of bone

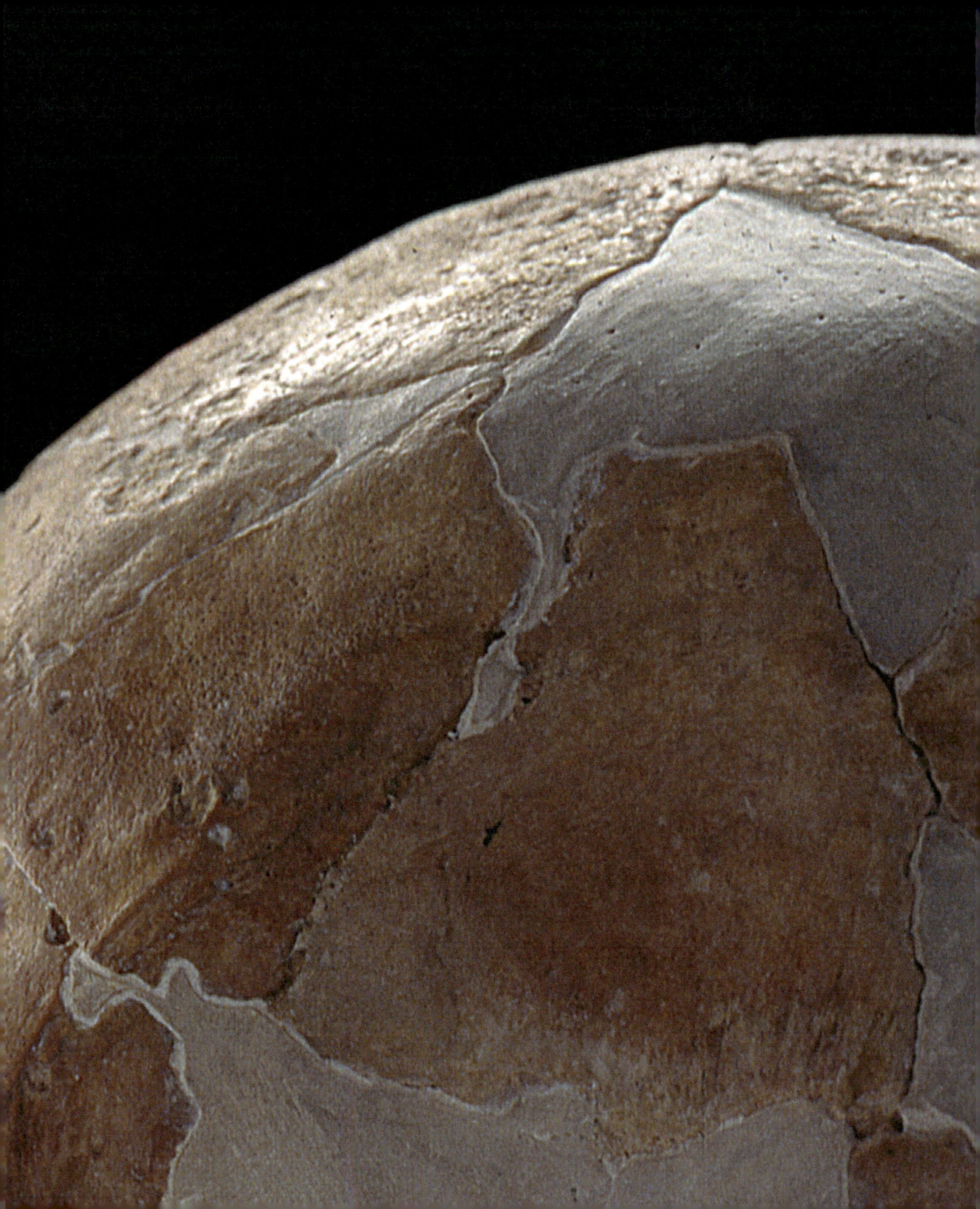

Contents

Contributors

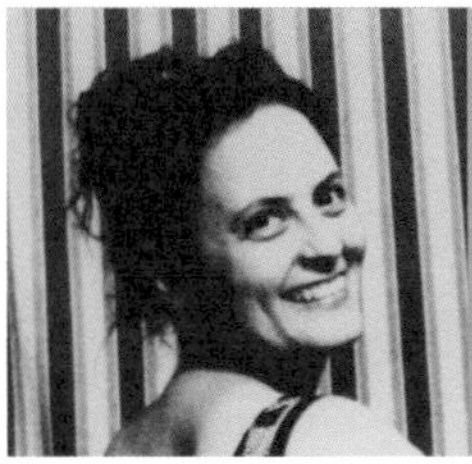

Joni Brenner is a principal tutor in History of Art at the Wits School of Arts, University of the Witwatersrand and a practising visual artist. She exhibits her work regularly both locally and in London.

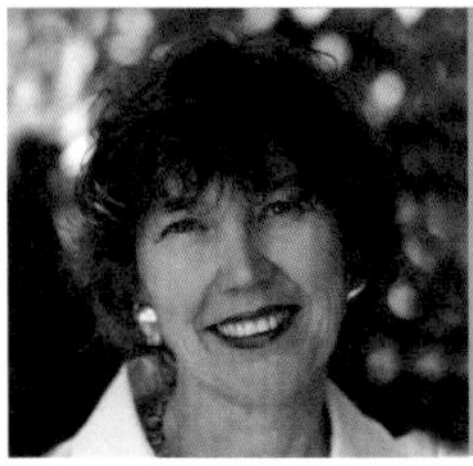

Elizabeth Burroughs is a senior manager at Umalusi. She has written twice previously on the work of Joni Brenner and edited several texts on visual artists including Karel Nel and Edoardo Villa.

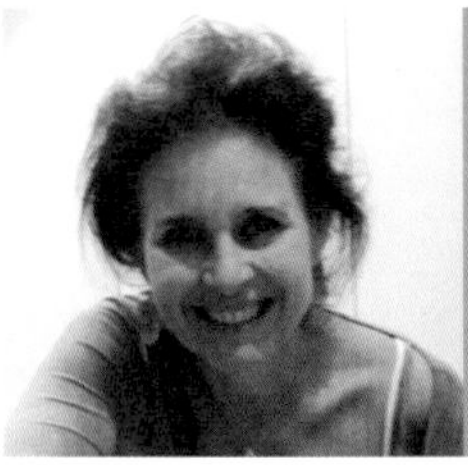

Debbie Glencross is an associate professor in the Department of Molecular Medicine and Haematology at Wits and the National Health Laboratory Service. Best known for her development of a novel affordable laboratory PLG CD4 test currently used in more than 100 laboratories across southern Africa, she is also an artist and printmaker.

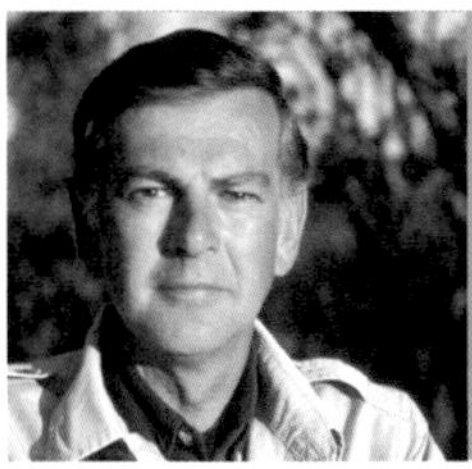

Donald Johanson is the founding director of the Institute of Human Origins at Arizona State University. He is best known for his discovery of Lucy, the 3.2-million-year-old skeleton from Ethiopia. A lively and controversial palaeoanthropologist, he is co-author of nine books, including *Lucy: The Beginnings of Humankind* (with Maitland Edey), *From Lucy to Language* (with Blake Edgar) and most recently, *Lucy's Legacy: The Quest for Human Origins*, (with Kate Wong).

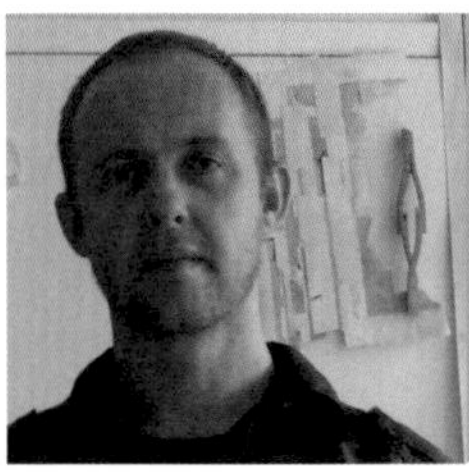

Gerhard Marx is an artist, theatre director and filmmaker, and has collaborated with a number of like-minded practitioners including Philip Miller, William Kentridge, Maja Marx, Lara Foot Newton, and the Handspring Puppet Company. He is represented by the Goodman Gallery.

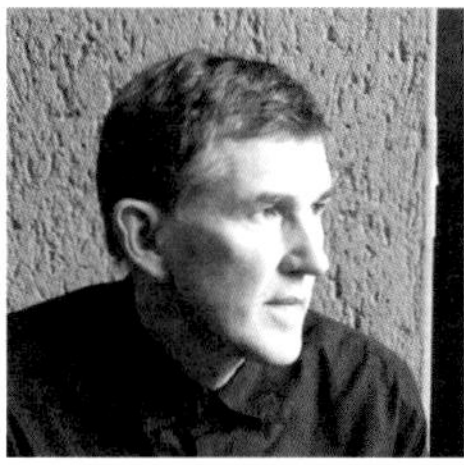

Karel Nel is an artist and an associate professor of Fine Arts at the Wits School of Arts. He is a respected collector of African, Asian and Oceanic art with a particular interest in currencies. He has expertise in southern African art and advises and consults with museums in South Africa, New York, London and Paris. Nel is artist-in-residence for COSMOS – an astronomy project mapping two degrees square of the universe.

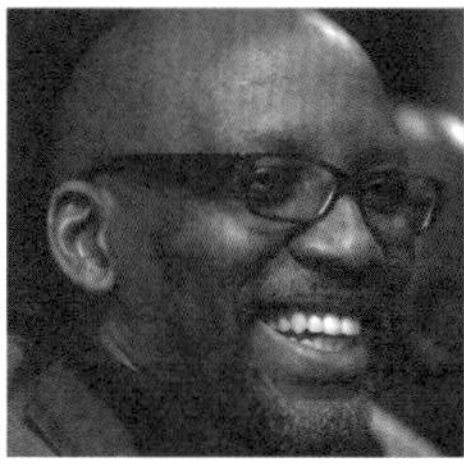

Kopano Ratele is a professor at the Institute for Social and Health Sciences at the University of South Africa. His insistence on probing the human psyche within its social and cultural context provides a powerful tool for understanding ourselves and is explored in his recent publication, *There was this goat*, co-written with Antjie Krog and Nosisi Mpolweni.

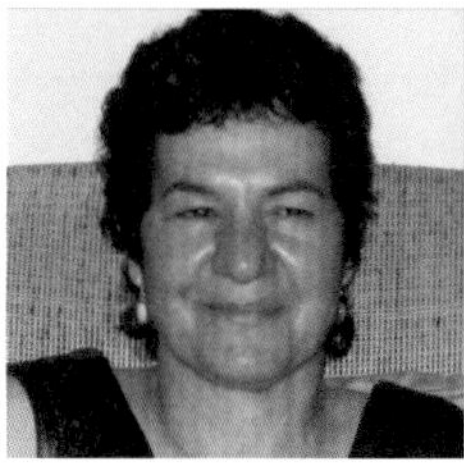

Lynne Slonimsky is a lecturer in Curriculum Studies at the School of Education at Wits. She has published in the areas of early reading instruction, pedagogy, assessment and curriculum policy. She is driven to write poetry on far too few occasions.

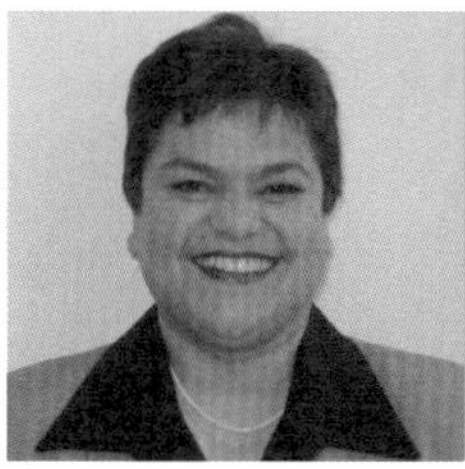

Himla Soodyall is an associate professor in the Department of Human Genetics at Wits, and the director of the Medical Research Council's Human Genomic Diversity and Diseases Research Unit, in partnership with Wits and the National Health Laboratory Services. A leading scholar in genetic diversity and human migratory patterns, Soodyall believes in the value of making complex scientific ideas accessible to non-scientists.

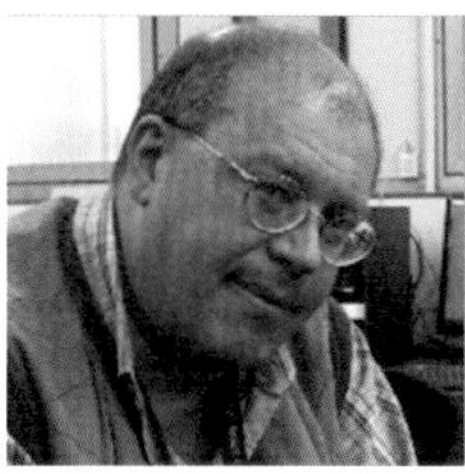

Bernhard Zipfel is a palaeoanthropologist with a special interest in the evolution of the human foot, the origins of hominin bipedalism and palaeopathology. He manages the fossil primate and non-primate collections housed at the Institute for Human Evolution and curates the fossil collections at the Bernard Price Institute for Palaeontological Research and the rock collections at the Wits School of Geosciences.

Acknowledgements

The making of this book and the exhibition it accompanies has been both a long and collaborative process of thinking, talking, reading, writing, making, planning, expanding and finally pulling it together into the form it is now.

The interdisciplinary terrain of the project has meant that the conversations that have informed its birth have been far-reaching and, at times, unfamiliar. Several institutes and individuals have supported our work, and without them, the project would not have been possible.

For their ideas, input and advice in the initial stages of conceptualising the project, we thank Francis Thackeray, director of the Institute of Human Evolution (IHE), Geoff Blundell, director of the Origins Centre and Andrea Leenen, director of the Palaeontological Scientific Trust (PAST). We gratefully acknowledge their support throughout the development of the project. Tawana Kupe, Dean of the Wits Faculty of Humanities, has read various drafts of essays and proposals, and his enthusiastic belief in our work has been inspiring. We thank Scott Hazelhurst for his comments and insights on nearly all the stages of the manuscript. Belinda Bozzoli, Deputy-Vice Chancellor for Research, embraced our project and enabled its fruition at a critical point in its financial life, and we thank her deeply. We also thank Georges Pfruender, head of the Wits School of Arts, for his support. Julie Miller and Veronica Klipp at Wits University Press believed in this project and undertook with great professionalism to see it through to publication under tight deadline pressures. We are grateful for their courage in supporting a strange hybrid book that seeks to dispel polarities between art and science. Ruksana Osman and several of her staff from the School of Education have also seen the potential value of a multimodal project such as this for research, teaching and learning at school and tertiary levels and we warmly acknowledge their role in using this exhibition and publication in diverse contexts. We thank Lee Berger and Bonita de Klerk for facilitating the particular way in which the Taung fossil is displayed and Lee Berger for the loan of a high security display cabinet for the Taung fossil. Standard Bank is acknowledged for the loan of cabinets to display the Border Cave 1 specimen and the modern chimpanzee skull. Of course, we are extremely grateful to the Wits Hominin Access Advisory Committee for loaning us the fossils themselves. We extend warm thanks to the two anonymous peer reviewers whose comments and insights significantly helped to improve the manuscript. Kevin Shenton and Karel Nel are acknowledged for their inspired design of the book, Vanessa Perlman for her intelligent and sharp copy-editing and Ethné Clarke for indexing this book. We thank the Adler Museum of Medicine and the many photographers and archivists who agreed to let us use their images. They are individually acknowledged on the copyrights page. John Hodgkiss, Michael Hall, Bob Cnoops, Abrie Fourie and Clive Hassall are thanked for their beautiful photography of the artists' works. Joni Brenner and Karel Nel thank ArtFirst, London, and Gerhard Marx thanks the Goodman Gallery, South Africa for their support, the Warren Siebrits Collection and The Marvellous Collection for the loan of artworks. Karel Nel extends sincere thanks to Ron Clarke, Morris Sutton, Sarah Roberts and Mark Behr for making the collection of site-specific dusts possible. We thank the Origins Centre team, Fred Glick and Peter Mitchell, for the installation of the exhibition. Finally, we are deeply grateful to PAST, IHE, the Vice-Chancellor's Office at Wits and the Strategic Planning Division who collectively funded this project.

Joni Brenner
Elizabeth Burroughs
Debbie Glencross
Don Johanson
Gerhard Marx
Karel Nel
Kopano Ratele
Lynne Slonimsky
Himla Soodyall
Bernhard Zipfel

May 2011

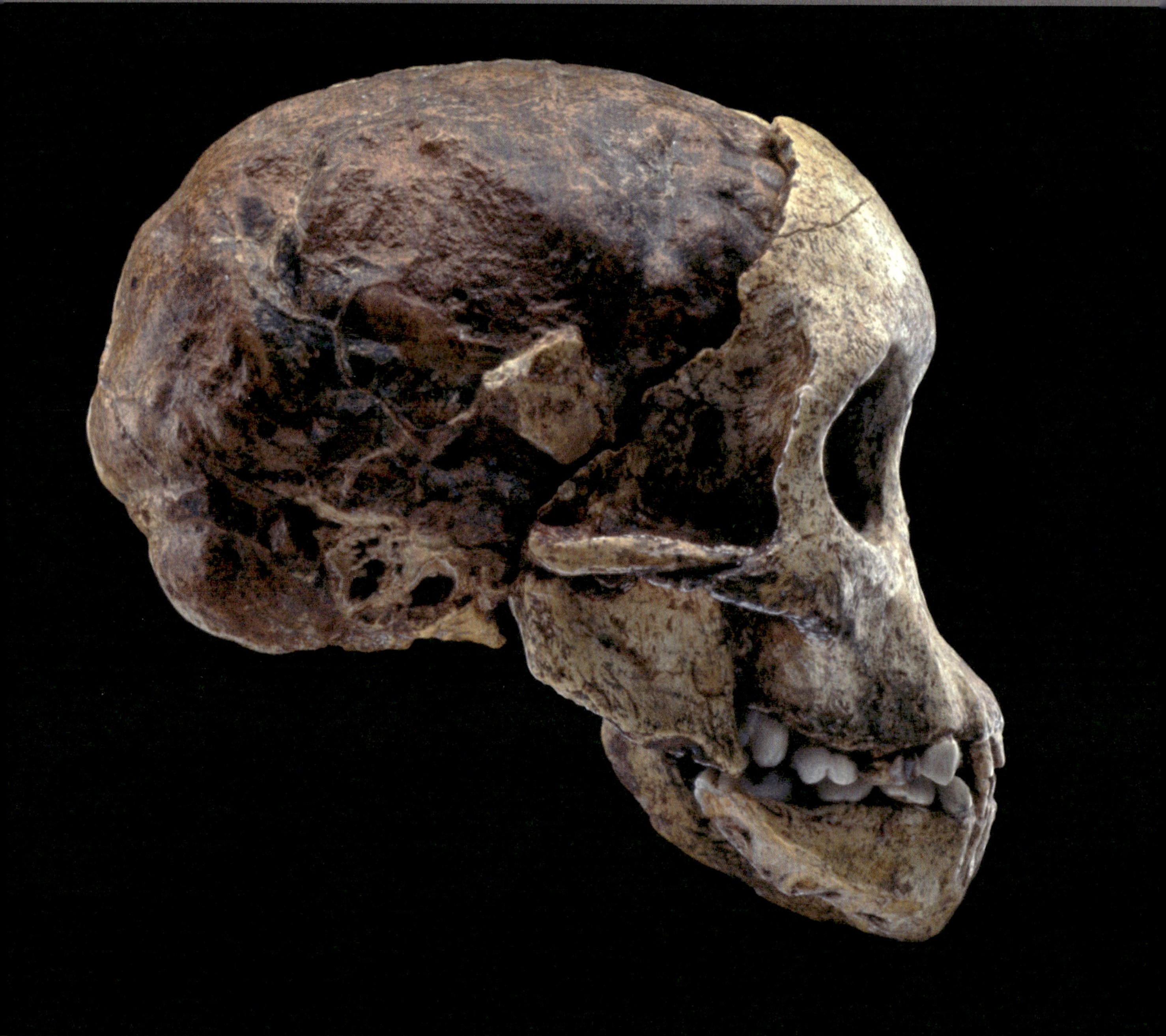

Foreword

Bernhard Zipfel

The *Life of bone* exhibition and the publication of this book coincide with the 85th anniversary of the discovery of the Taung skull at the Buxton Limeworks near Taung in what is now the North West Province. In 1924, Raymond Dart, an anatomist from the University of the Witwatersrand, recognised that the skull, still embedded in a solid breccia matrix, was different from anything he had seen before – undoubtedly a higher primate but neither monkey nor modern human. He finally called it *Australopithecus africanus* – or southern ape of Africa – and suggested that, even though the fossilised skull was similar to that of an ape, it belonged to a species that had taken steps well along the road to humanity. With the exception of support from Robert Broom and a few others, the broader scientific community foolishly repudiated Dart's revolutionary proposal until after 1950. For 25 years after the discovery, the significance of this remarkable find was fiercely disputed. At that time, the so-called Piltdown man was considered to be an early hominin,[1] suggesting that humans evolved in England and Europe in the Pleistocene. By 1953, it was evident that the Piltdown skull was a hoax, and attention was finally turned to the Taung skull. Only then was Dart's assertion vindicated. Finally, in 1984, the journal *Science* included the Taung child and Dart's interpretation of it as one of 20 scientific discoveries that shaped the life of humans in the 20th century.

Australopithecus africanus, Taung, Sterkfontein, skull, lateral right. Photograph by David Brill, 1985, Faculty of Health Sciences, University of the Witwatersrand.

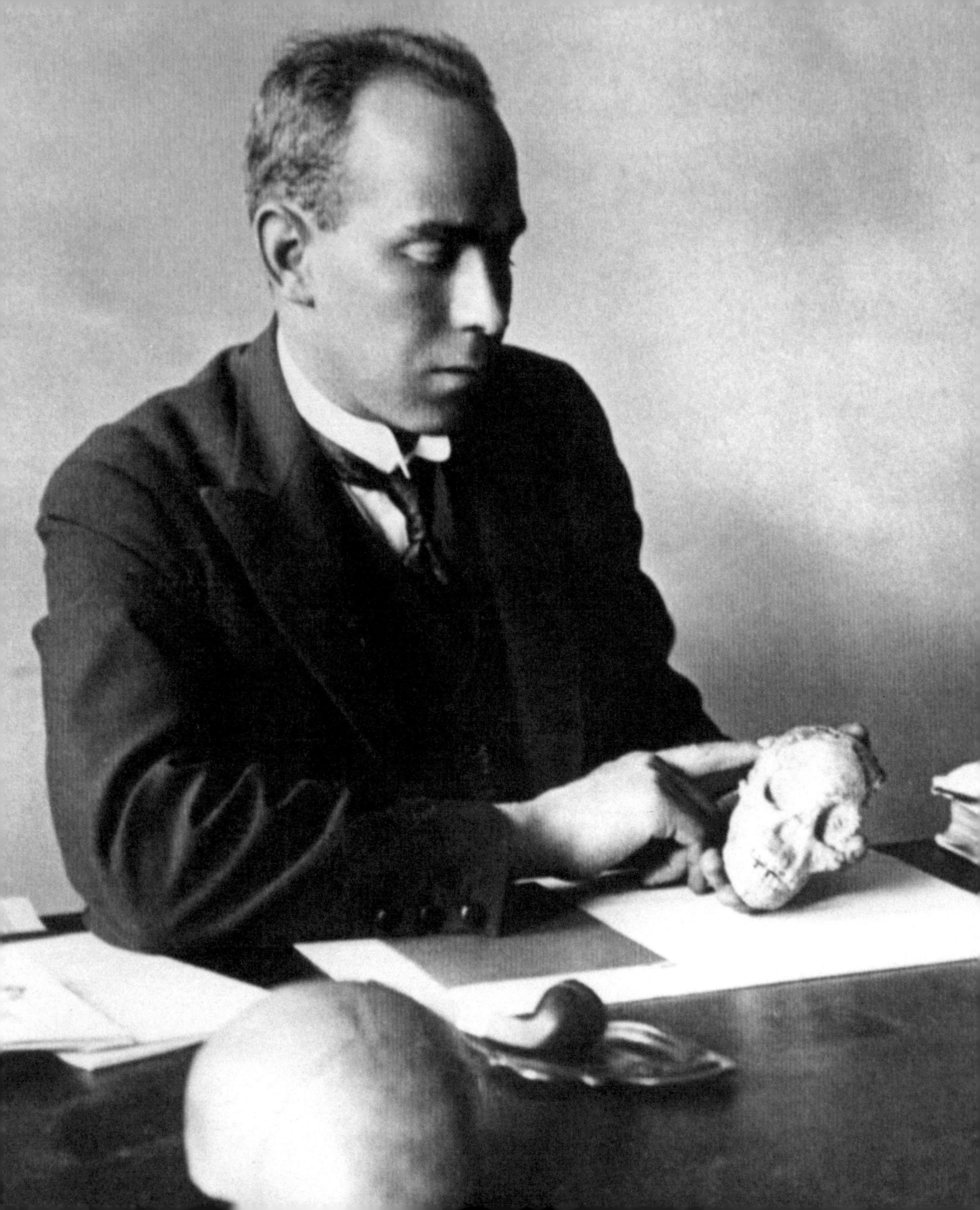

LEFT: Raymond Dart, 1925. Photograph courtesy Barlow Rand and Phillip Tobias.

TOP RIGHT: *Australopithecus africanus*, Taung, Sterkfontein, skull, 3/4 right. Photograph by David Brill, 1985, courtesy Faculty of Health Sciences, University of the Witwatersrand.

BOTTOM RIGHT: *Pan troglodytes* (chimpanzee), skull, 3/4 right. Photograph by Ted Thai, 2002, courtesy Museum of Natural History, NYC /Getty Images.

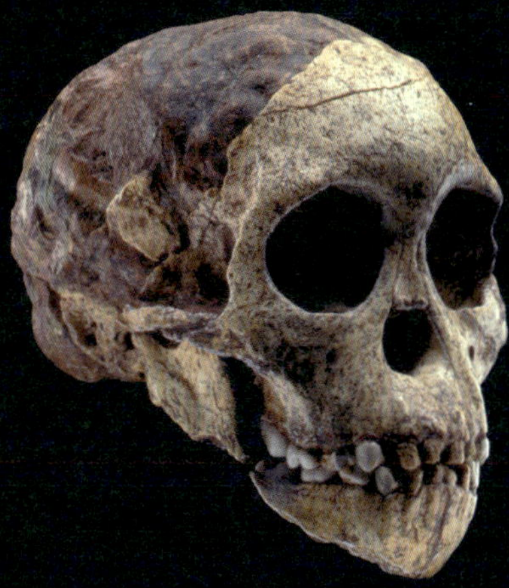

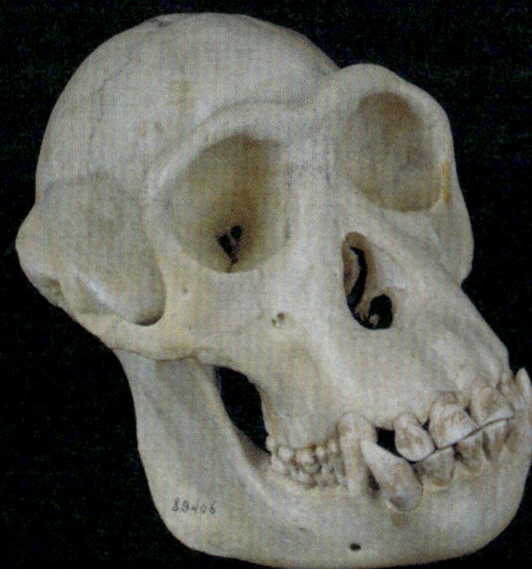

As curator of fossils, I am privileged to be one of the very few people who regularly have the opportunity to see and handle the Taung child's skull. When I show the skull to both scientists and non-scientists, the almost predictable expressions of wonder are clearly not only brought about by the scientific significance of this, the type specimen of *Australopithecus africanus*, but also by the sheer beauty of the little skull. How can this be? Surely the remains of a dead creature cannot be 'beautiful'? Well, here we have the well-preserved, fossilised remains of a skull of a long extinct creature reminiscent of both humans and apes. It consists of the face of a child of about three, the lower jaw with its perfectly preserved teeth and, remarkably, also the brain endocast formed by sediments that partially filled the inside of the cranium. In the process of fossilisation over a period of approximately 2.5 million years, other minerals replaced the bone, and calcite crystals formed on the brain endocast, like stalagmites in a miniature cave. This has resulted in a subtle patina that, when carefully examined, shows delicate detail of anatomy in various shades of colour, enhancing every marking on the skull. One can only think of it as beautiful, both in terms of its scientific importance – it being the very first early hominin discovered – and its aesthetic characteristics so reminiscent of a work of art. It evokes emotion in those who see it. I experience gooseflesh every time I carefully pick it up.

Border Cave 1 cranium of *Homo sapiens*, lateral left.
Photograph by Dr Gerald Newlands, 1992, courtesy of
Faculty of Health Sciences, University of the Witwatersrand.

The second skull on display is known as the Border Cave 1 skull, found on the border between South Africa and Swaziland. Being at least 71 000 years old, and possibly as old as 171 000 years before present, this skull is a rare example of an early anatomically modern human, and one of the earliest examples of a person who looked like people living today. When studying sub-fossil or fossilised pre-historic, anatomically modern humans from southern Africa, the similarities to the Taung skull are inescapable. A similar fossilisation process has taken place, and though the Border Cave remains may be fragmentary, the facial features can be recognised as human, even by the uninformed. The Border Cave 1 skull belonged to one of those early pre-pastoralists whose voices were the first human ones to be heard on this continent.

The third skull is that of a chimpanzee, one of the African Great Apes, which, in his contemplation of the origin of the human species, led Darwin to conclude that humans would have evolved in Africa. The three specimens displayed as part of the *Life of bone* project thus present a compacted trajectory of a section of the evolutionary model. The lineages of modern humans and *Australopithecus africanus* are thought to have diverged roughly 2.5 million years ago, and 2.5 million years before that, their common lineage split from that of the chimpanzee. One marvels at the way nature, by means of the evolutionary process of natural

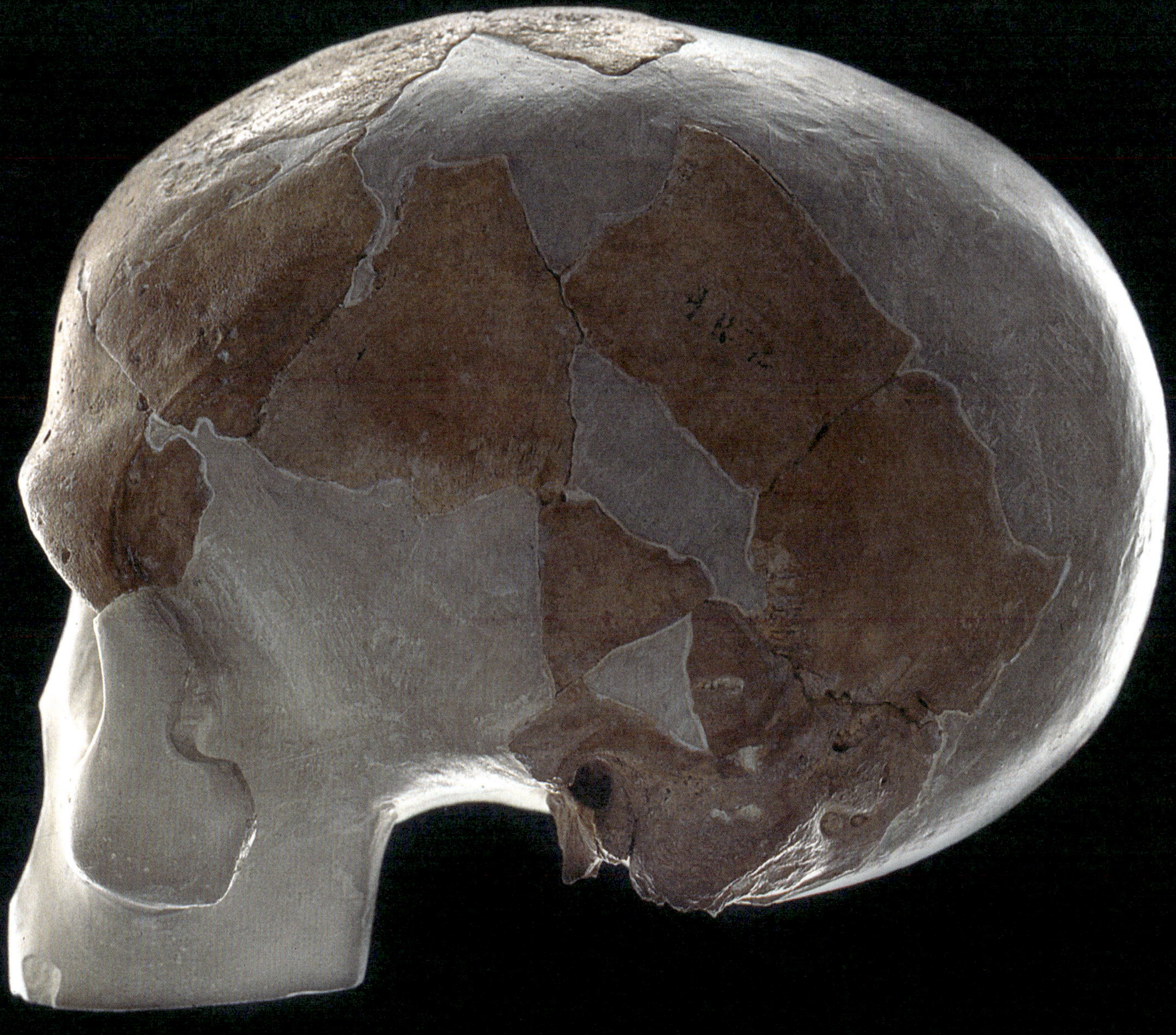

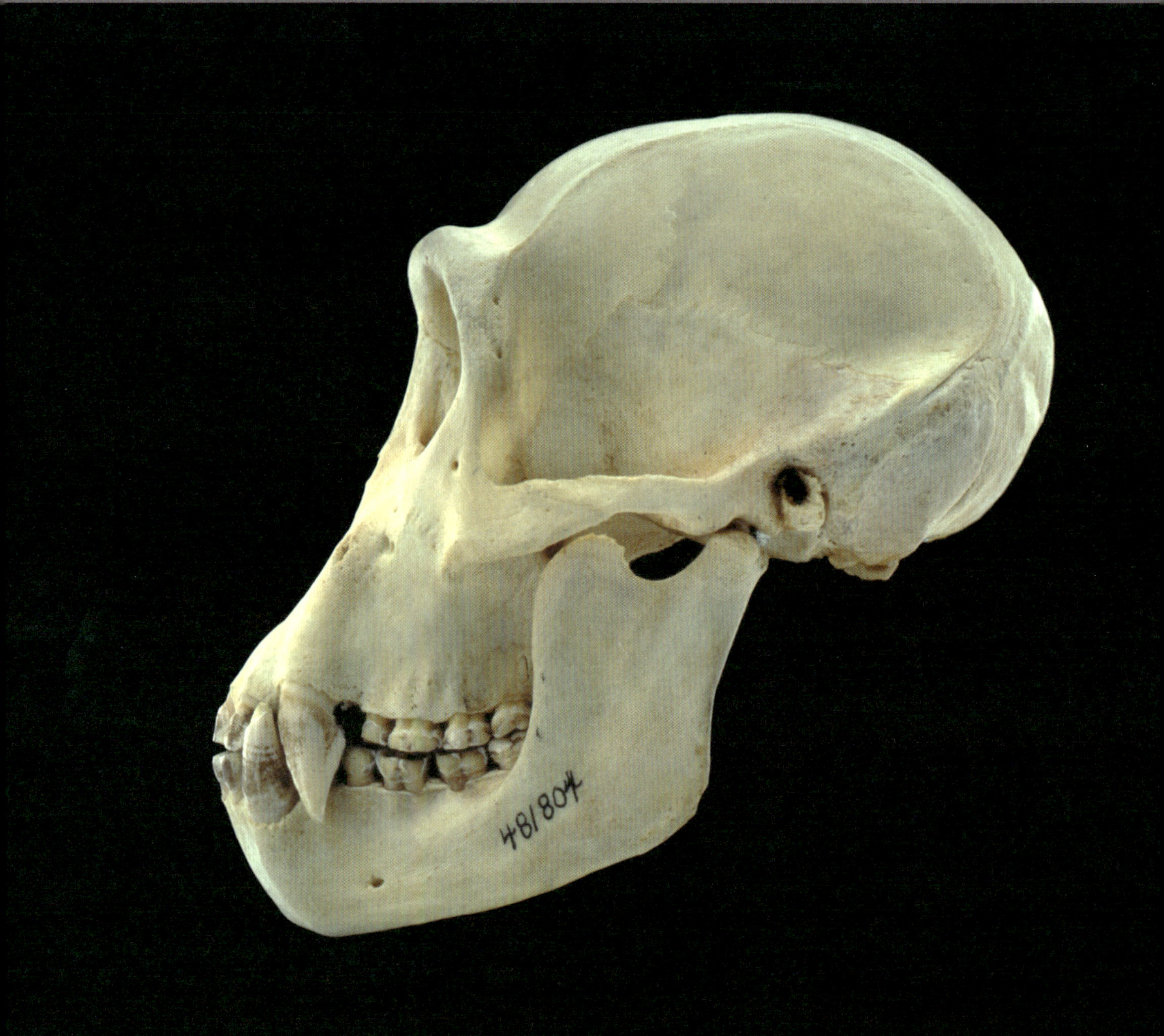
481804

Pan troglodytes, male (chimpanzee), skull, lateral left. Photograph by David Brill, 1996, courtesy Division of Mammals, National Museum of Natural History (NMNH), Smithsonian Institution.

selection, has brought us to where we are today. Taken together, the three skulls represent some of the terrain of enquiry in this project.

Life of bone has deliberately set out to consider the relationship between science and art. A group of prominent artists and scientists has used the fossils as the focus for dialogue. Through their various explorations, the group encourages us to access a more intimate side of our impressions of and responses to the Taung skull. Scientists are challenged to appreciate an alternative form of interpretation of the fossils they work with. Artists are impelled to reflect on the significance of science in society. Above all, the *Life of bone* project provides an opportunity to use science and art to translate our history into forms that engage the general viewer, which, we hope, will encourage public interest in our unique heritage.

Bernhard Zipfel
Curator of Collections
University of the Witwatersrand

Notes

1 Hominid refers to the group consisting of all modern and extinct Great Apes (that is, modern humans, chimpanzees, gorillas and orang-utans plus all their immediate ancestors). The terms hominid and hominin are often used interchangeably, but hominin is a more specific term that refers only to living humans, extinct human species and all our immediate ancestors (including members from the genera *Homo*, *Australopithecus*, *Paranthropus* and *Ardipithecus*).

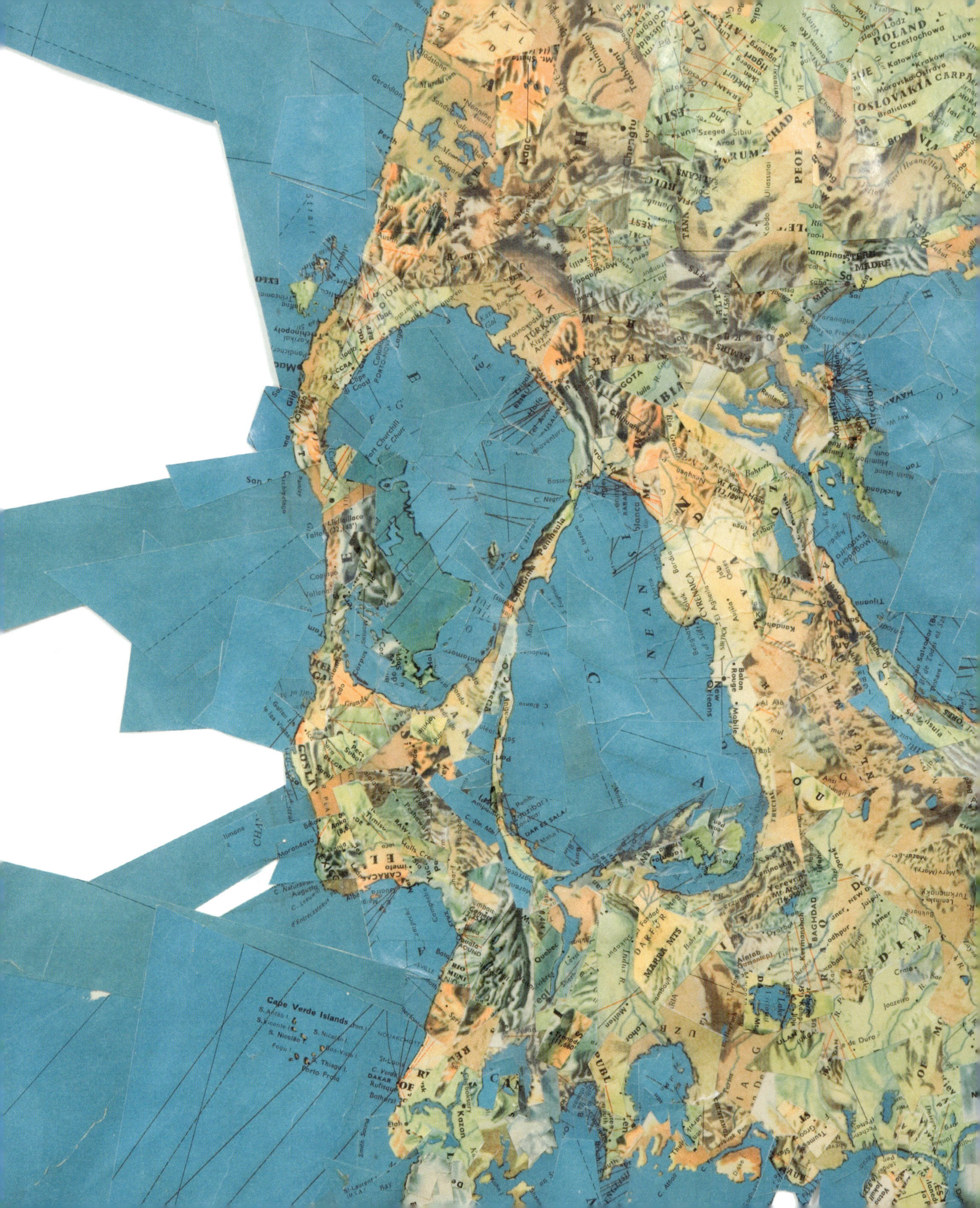

POLAND
Cape Verde Islands
BAGHDAD
MARRA MTS
New Orleans
CARACAS

Chapter 1

Obsessions and impulses: art meets science

Joni Brenner, Elizabeth Burroughs, Debbie Glencross

In an article in *New Scientist*, art historian Martin Kemp reflects on the current separation or severance between art and science. He comments that many intelligent, motivated people are interested in art and science but find that much art doesn't relate to their lives, and that a great deal of science is mightily obscure.[1]

The genesis of *Life of bone*

The *Life of bone* project, an exhibition and this accompanying book, began as conversations between three contemporary South African artists – Joni Brenner, Gerard Marx and Karel Nel – whose practices over many years, directly and indirectly, have included the consideration of bones, human and fossil, in their making. In their artistic explorations these artists have dealt with issues of human origin, evolution, deep time, lineage, ancestry and belonging. Conversations, which often took place in the presence of skeletal remains and the casts of hominid fossils, reflected on ways of knowing, mapping and telling; on things we can and cannot know about our histories; and on the natural and social forces that have an impact on how we understand these material remains and ourselves.

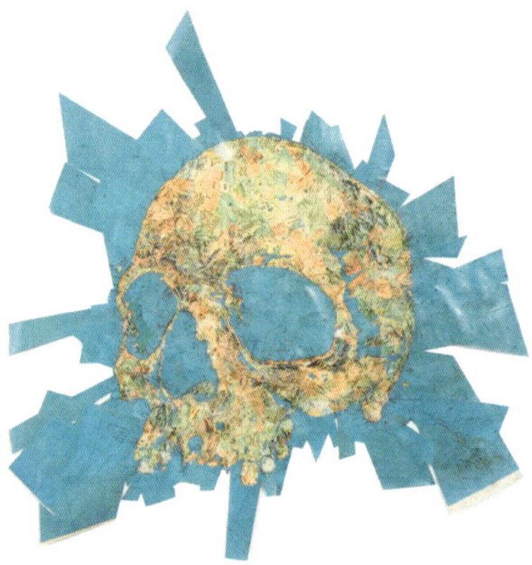

Gerhard Marx, *Aggregate Skull 1*, cut and reconstituted map fragments, 123.5 x 123.5 cm (detail left), 2010.

From quite early on, in conceptualising this project, the three artists began talking to scientists, writers and people interested in osteology, in what bones can and cannot tell us, in research and in ways of representing knowledge. All are people interested in exploring the limitations of their own disciplines. The conversations broadened to include individuals who are multiply researchers, scientists (palaeoanthropologists, geneticists, pathologists), guardians of archives of cultural objects (bones and artworks), educators, writers and socio-cultural scholars. Part of the novelty of the *Life of bone* project is the cross-disciplinary reach of the conversations that have shaped the exhibition, and the ways in which the visual and textual investigations can be viewed as directed practice towards the 'evidence'. This book presents some of the art-science encounters among the participants in the build-up to the exhibition.

Much of the discussion among us has centred on the scientific and evolutionary significance of the Taung fossil, especially in respect of how its discovery challenged conventional wisdom about the origin of the human lineage and provided support for Darwin's proposition that humankind had its origins in Africa. Raymond Dart's interpretation of the fossil skull discovered at Taung disrupted the accepted construction of knowledge and, for that reason, was received with hostility. We considered the critical relationship between new evidence and its impact on the body of accepted scientific opinion, and how similar it was to the reception of a radically new paradigm in art when the influence of an African aesthetic found its way into the work of Picasso and his contemporaries.

We thought about how each fossil discovery is interpreted in relation to existing fossils and, very often, discoveries fundamentally change what we know, resulting in shifts to the location of existing fossils within the model. Science proceeds precisely when anomalies are resolved and knowledge moves into a new paradigm, with its own sets of anomalies and missing information. It is in this way, through engagement with the past, that the past itself is in constant flux.

Artistic exploration also proceeds through active dialogues with other artists across time and place, building on existing models and overturning and/or reinventing them on the way. T.S. Eliot asserts that the past should be altered by the present as much as the present is directed by the past[2] and Michael Baxandall writes that 'if one says that X influenced Y it does seem that one is saying that X did something to Y rather than Y did something to X. But in the consideration of good pictures and painters the second is always the more lively reality'[3] and Mieke Bal has done much work around the idea that art's engagement with what came before it involves an active reworking of existing models.[4] Building on Bal's proposition, Norman Bryson writes in his essay entitled, "Bacon's dialogues with the past" that 'although Bacon stated that his paintings were "after" Velasquez, perhaps we can turn the proposition around: what is Velasquez after Bacon?' Bryson's investigation unpacks the possibility that the latter artist *produces* the earlier one through a 'preposterous' logic of reversed influence.[5] What this line of thinking does is negate the one-way street or linear process of knowledge construction. In showing how the present shapes the past as much as the past shapes the present, it dispels any notions of a static past, and shows how a dialectical relationship across time and place brings renewed and contemporary significance to things from the recent or ancient past. One of the aims of *Life of bone* is to re-see, in a sense, the Taung fossil, and by extension other palaeontological and historical material in terms of the present. How do the visual and textual responses to issues arising from the material presence of these fossils prompt a re-seeing of the past and of the present? How is it useful to think about what bones do and do not tell us?

Life of bone: the ways of knowing

In finding the title for the exhibition and book, *Life of bone,* it was as if many of the disparate thoughts we had entertained suddenly coalesced. Elizabeth Hallam's[6] reference to 'the diverse post-mortem lives of bones' encapsulates the paradox that we had been engaged with – that bones are both dead and yet live. Hallam observes how bones' salience is determined by their examination in social contexts, and the idea that their meaning is, in her words, unstable. In all our discussions, we were recognising that the life of bones is dependent on their being intellectually contextualised and re-contextualised. For humankind, bones inescapably become the focus of different kinds of conjecture and meaning-making. This capacity to think about bones and to be deeply affected by them, this desire to understand their identity, is a distinguishing feature of what it means to be human. As Kopano Ratele writes: 'To become part of a culture, discipline, or project, bones need interpreters – palaeontologists, painters, sculptors, kin. Stories must be told about them.'

During the process of engagement, the discussions which had begun with ancient fossil bones and the physical remains of persons whose identities were unknown and irretrievable, the inclusion of Himla Soodyall and Kopano Ratele in the discussion brought a more contemporary cast to the *Life of bone* project, with their interests in and involvement with the TRC hearings and the return of the remains of Sarah Bartmann.

So, in the course of the project, the team has considered some of the ways in which people have endeavoured to contextualise, and so understand bones.

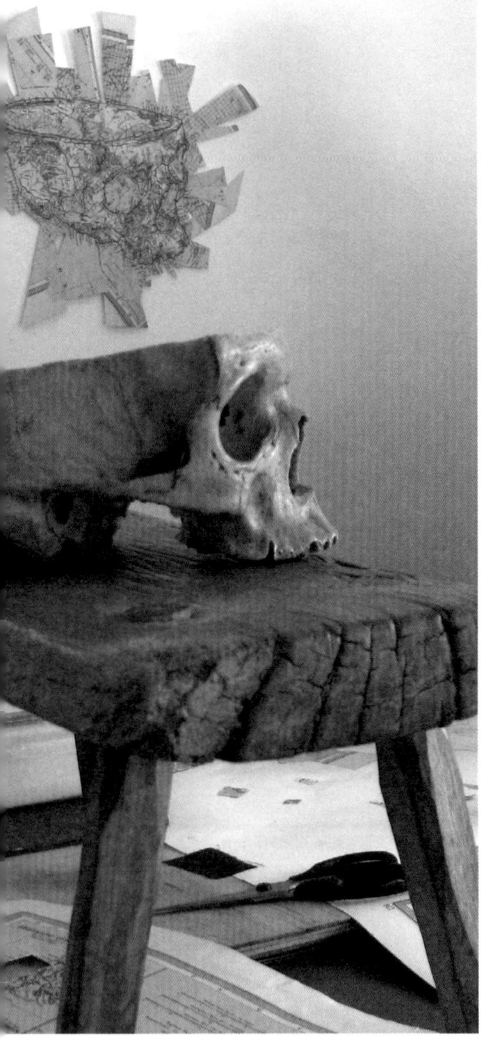

Geology

Early hominin and hominid fossils are, on their discovery, placed on a timeline in accordance with a geological understanding of the site. The dating of the Taung skull to approximately 2.5 million years ago is related to geological interpretation of its location in the Buxton Limeworks breccias. Early fossils such as the Leakey finds in Olduvai, which have eroded out of surrounding rock due to their exceptional hardness, mean that the reliable data about these bones resides in their physical location in rock strata. This impersonal context, the isolated nature of the finds, the transformation of bone into stone, and the 'otherness' of these very early skeletal remains allow for a more dispassionate relationship with the bones. Contemporary artist, Hiroshi Sugimoto, has observed that fossils are 'the earliest photographs', reproductions of an original moment in distant time. What this statement reminds us is that the original bone of the fossil has long since been displaced, and they are thus already representations of the original.

Taphonomy

Taphonomy is the science that explores how and why organisms are preserved, as well as the study of the spatial relations between finds within a particular site. People who study fossilised remains use taphonomy to understand how fossils form and what might have created gaps in the fossil record: soft tissues, for example, do not generally survive fossilisation, and the rare endocranial cast of the Taung skull, which preserves the brain structure, is a remarkable exception. Taphonomy, a word which means 'the laws of burial' is a science that studies the processes of death, decay and preservation, and is often used forensically to understand the context of the find.

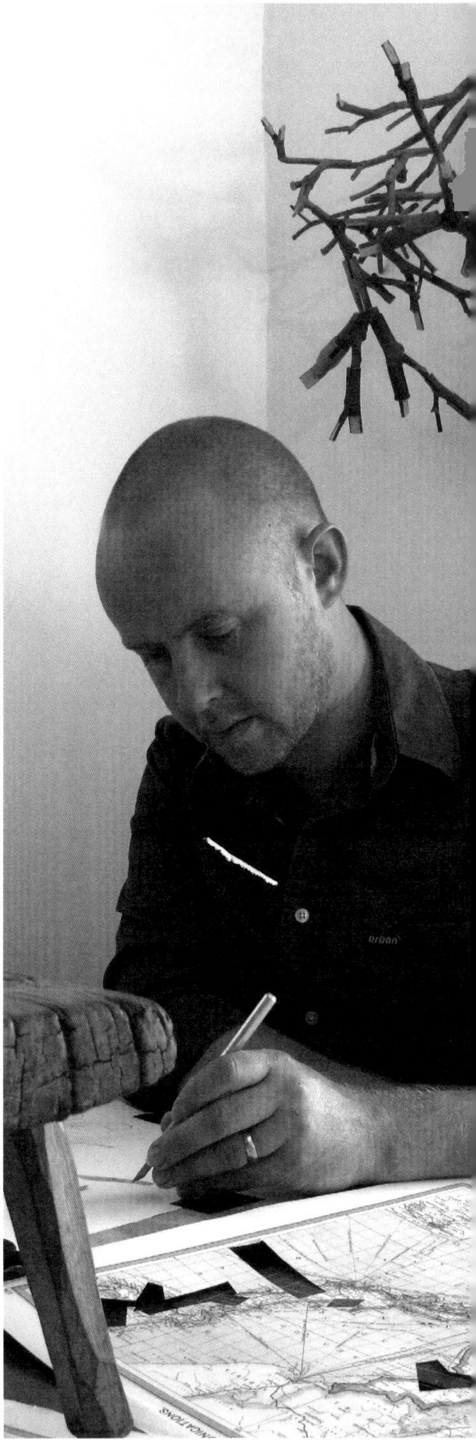

Comparative anatomy

One of the primary means of relating fossil finds to one another occurs through a comparison of their anatomical structures. The result of an anatomical analysis, a process that can take decades, leads to the description of the fossil type. As Roger Lewin points out repeatedly in his book, *Bones of contention,*[7] where the evidence is limited, the interpretation has greater prominence. Lewin never forgets that hominid fossil discoveries always involve both the self-image of humanity and that of individual scientists. Donald Johanson reinforces this notion when he calls palaeoanthropologists the most argumentative kind of *sapiens.*

In recent years, comparative anatomy has looked back far beyond the hominin record to try to understand the biological relatedness across species. Johanson's plea for the protection of the higher apes is argued on the grounds of their sharing 99% of their DNA with humans.

Archaeology

Archaeology is the study of human societies through the recovery and analysis of the material culture and environmental data left behind. It frequently deals with older societies without a written record. Once one makes the move from the palaeoanthropological to the archaeological, a different form of ethics comes into play: the impact of finding a burial site where it is evident that a body has been deliberately interred is radically different from discovering fossils where there is no cultural context. In the team's discussions, the idea that evidence of a deliberate burial marks the presence of human consciousness has been much debated.

PAGES 12 AND 13: Gerhard Marx in his Melville studio, Johannesburg. Photograph by Maja Marx, 2011.

The evidence of care of the body after death seems to suggest the awareness of relationships and the need to protect the body from unwanted dissipation. It also suggests an awareness of past and future states, which in turn, suggests the possibility of self-reflection.

In addition to these identifiable disciplines, other more contemporary ones also lay claim to interpreting bones. In Chapter 2, Soodyall discusses the contribution made by DNA analysis to our understanding of human origins, while Ratele's work in Chapter 4 chimes with the enquiries of the Bones Collective research network, which emerged in social anthropology at the University of Edinburgh. The Collective's work is sampled in a special edition of the *Journal of Material Culture*, entitled "The substance of bones: the emotive materiality and affective presence of human remains".[8]

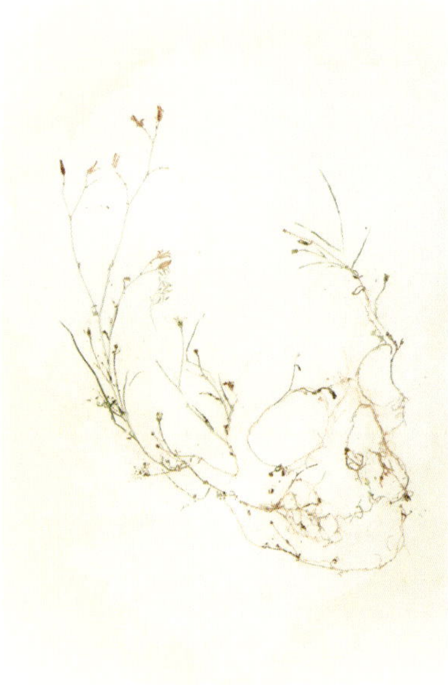

Gerhard Marx, *Skull 3*, plant material, acrylic paint and glue on cotton paper, 76 x 58 cm, (detail right), 2011

From the perspective of the team who has put together this book, the investigation of the meaning of bones also emerges from the discipline of art-making. The repeated analysis of a skull or a femur in the creative process gives rise to existential questions in much the same way as the interrogations undertaken by social anthropologists and scientists. It was heartening to find the drawings made at the *What lies beneath?* workshop, hosted by the Bones Collective in 2008, and to recognise the similarity of the questions that art-making prompts.

Structure of the book

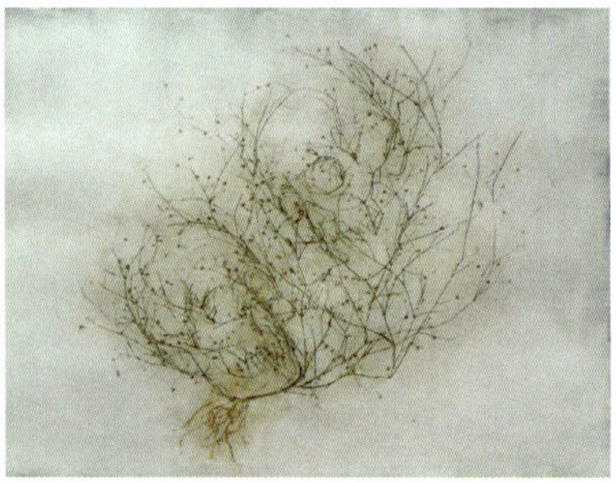

Gerhard Marx, *Father Father/Mother Mother*, plant matter, glue and watercolour on cotton paper, 57 x 75.5 cm, 2008.

This introductory essay establishes the scope of the project and points to its most central concerns. This chapter is followed by Soodyall's account of her experiences of working with human tissue to trace the divergence of distinct populations from a single, early African population through the DNA testing of living individuals. In the process, she considers Gerhard Marx's meditations on lineage. Chapter 3 deals with Marx's work and forms a companion piece to Chapters 5 and 8, where Elizabeth Burroughs writes in a mode that Joni Brenner has called 'creative non-fiction'. Chapters 4 and 5 are prompted by the work of Brenner, and include Ratele's thoughts on her painting and its relationship to South African

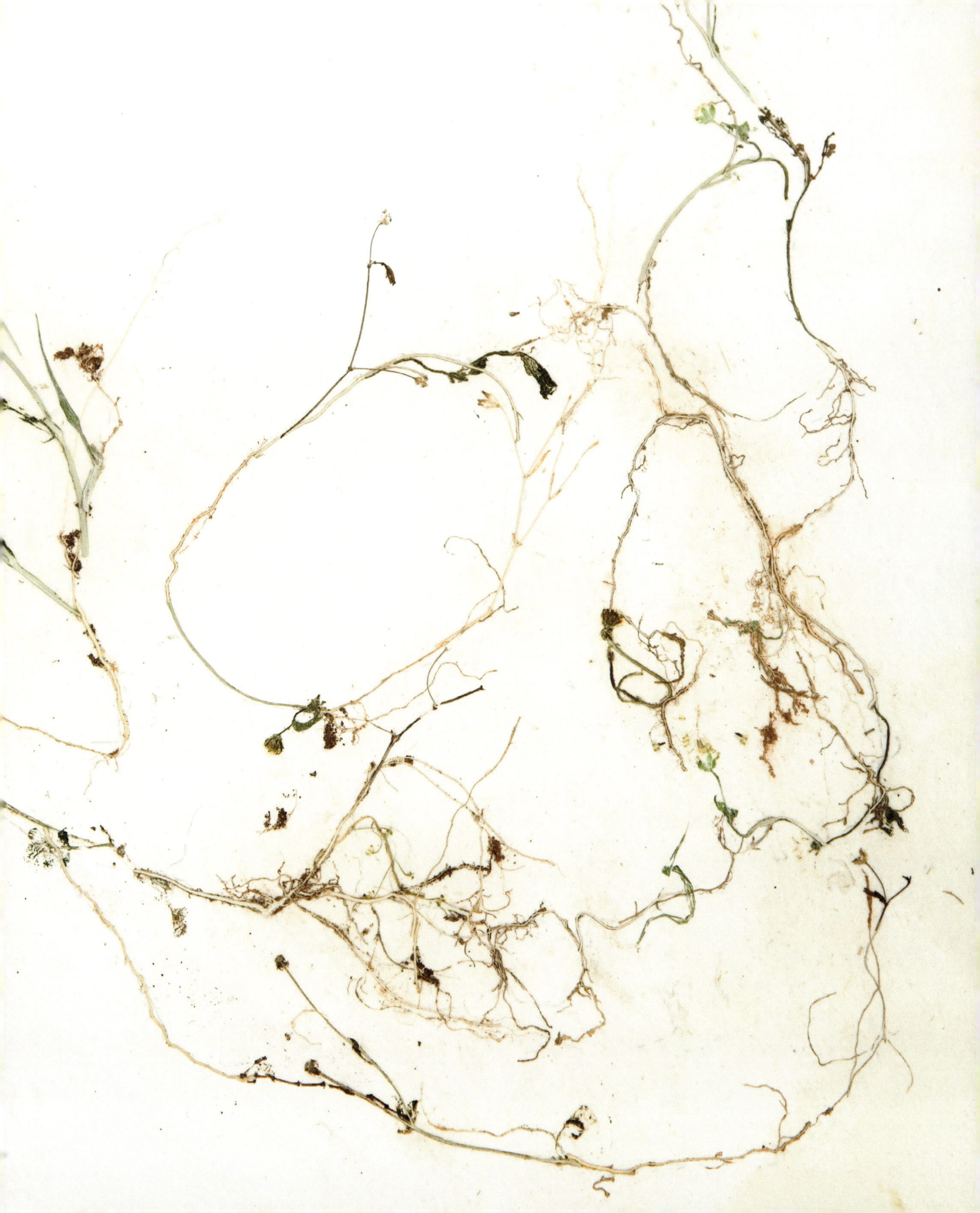

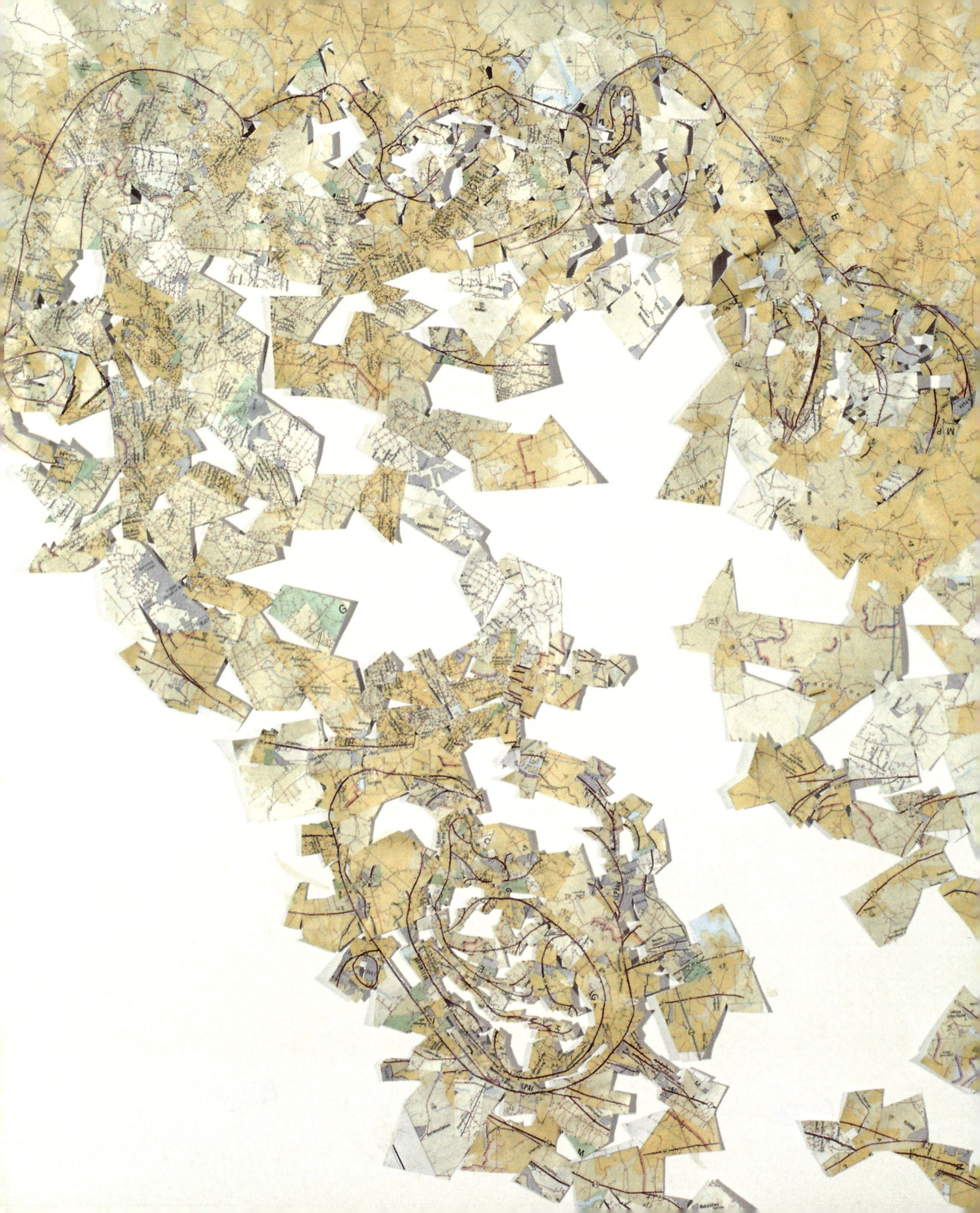

experiences of trauma. The final three chapters, chapter 6, 7 and 8, deal with the work of Karel Nel: the focus here lies in the nature of consciousness and his understanding of the overlaps in artistic and scientific enquiry. The book is rounded off by a short conclusion, which encapsulates some of the recurring concerns to emerge during the project. A poem by Lynne Slonimsky reactivates the affective nature of hominid bones.

A central passion in the *Life of bone* community is linking art and science to real-life concerns. In Soodyall's efforts to connect the role of DNA testing and studies in human genetics to learning about our lineages and location within patterns of evolution, she has used a comic-strip format. In adopting a story line that relates her scientific work to people's everyday realities, she anchors an understanding of scientific processes in both the public and individuals' consciousness.[9] Marx's visual register evokes deeply complex patterns of structure through which we locate ourselves in the world: rendering ideas and knowledge visually that Soodyall's own scientific research pursues in different ways. On the one hand, the organic materials Marx uses – roots and earth – are manipulated into images that appear diagrammatic with strong allusions to anatomical modes of representing information. On the other hand, Marx takes radically processed and inorganic forms like the arterial routes of a road atlas and cuts and splices them to create moving portraits of family members. These images of the human body are at once metaphorical anatomies of the impact of place and region on who we are, and emotional meditations on the traces and lines of connection between people – physical, emotional, geographical and genetic.

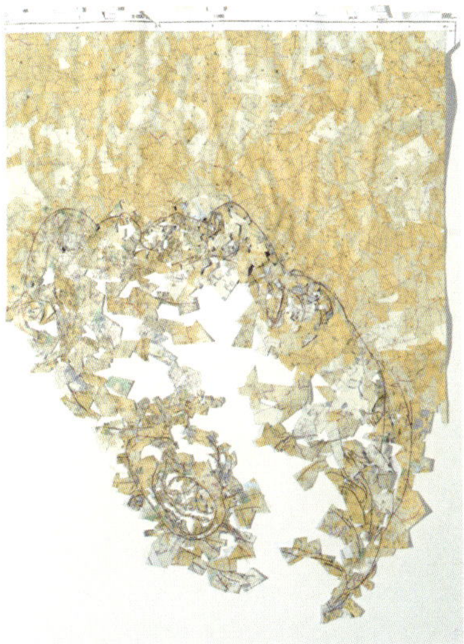

Gerhard Marx, *Sheet #2: head and portrait*, cut and reconstituted map fragments, 77 x 105 cm (detail left), 2005. UNISA Collection.

Life of bone has also attracted people whose work strives to demystify the sometimes obscure artistic and scientific processes so that things that have become radically severed might be reunited.[10] For many years, Nel has explored the relationship between art and science, working closely with palaeontologists on the one hand, and astronomers on the other, consistently investigating the ways in which artists and scientists embrace, as he puts it, 'similar febrile strategies to engage their insights.'[11]

Even while art and science both entertain the relationship between the known and the unknown, between certainty and uncertainty, between the graspable and the elusive, scientific research is nonetheless designed to reduce ambiguity. Artistic exploration, on the other hand, embraces ambiguity and uses it to allow unresolved reflections and assertions of the many ways in which we do not and cannot know. For all of Johanson's rigorous scientific analysis of hominid fossils, he has often mused, with Nel, upon who these beings were, what they thought, and what they felt – a humble reflection on the gaps in knowledge. His writing about fossils is rooted in his profound understanding of the meaning or value of fossils in the public imagination:

> Hominid fossils touch a responsive chord in people everywhere, who seem to have an inherent drive to know their beginnings. We want to know what the fossils have to say to us. There seems to be a magic in the fossilized bones that transcends time ... Ultimately, our fascination with the study of human origins nourishes our need for exploration and for understanding both our uniqueness and our close link to the natural world.[12]

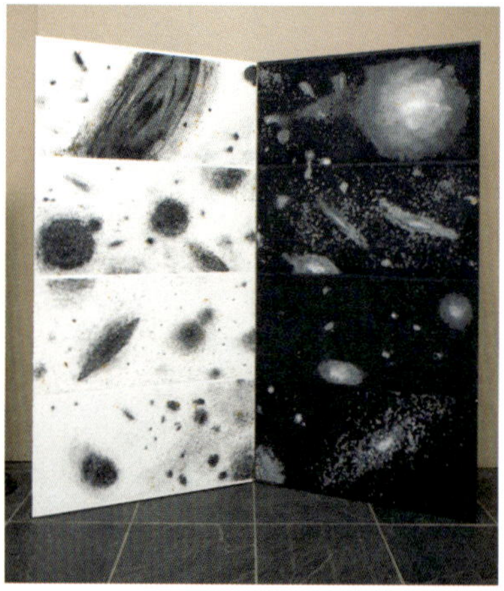

Karel Nel, *Galactic stratigraphy*, black carboniferous dust, salt, on wooden folding screen, 240 x 240 cm (detail right), 2009.

Johanson's essay in this book reflects on the relationship between nature and culture and on the combination of creative and destructive forces that our species embodies, ideas also central to Nel's work.

Both specific and abstract, Nel's work has the cool distance of forensic record yet is emotionally significant in content. He presents sheer fields of compacted dust collected from significant sites around the world – sites that have come to signal place/home, brutal socio-political moments in history or significant moments in scientific/evolutionary development. These juxtapositions are exemplified by the four new artworks Nel analyses in Chapter 7. Nel's work presents a distinctive and powerful combination of the conceptual and the physical, and engages the interface between experience/thought and its notation in visual form. His work as artist-in-residence on the COSMOS project – an astronomical survey of two degrees square of the universe – has meant that, whether working with palaeontologists or with astronomers, he is engaged with a visual mapping of scientific explorations towards understanding the origins of humankind, and of

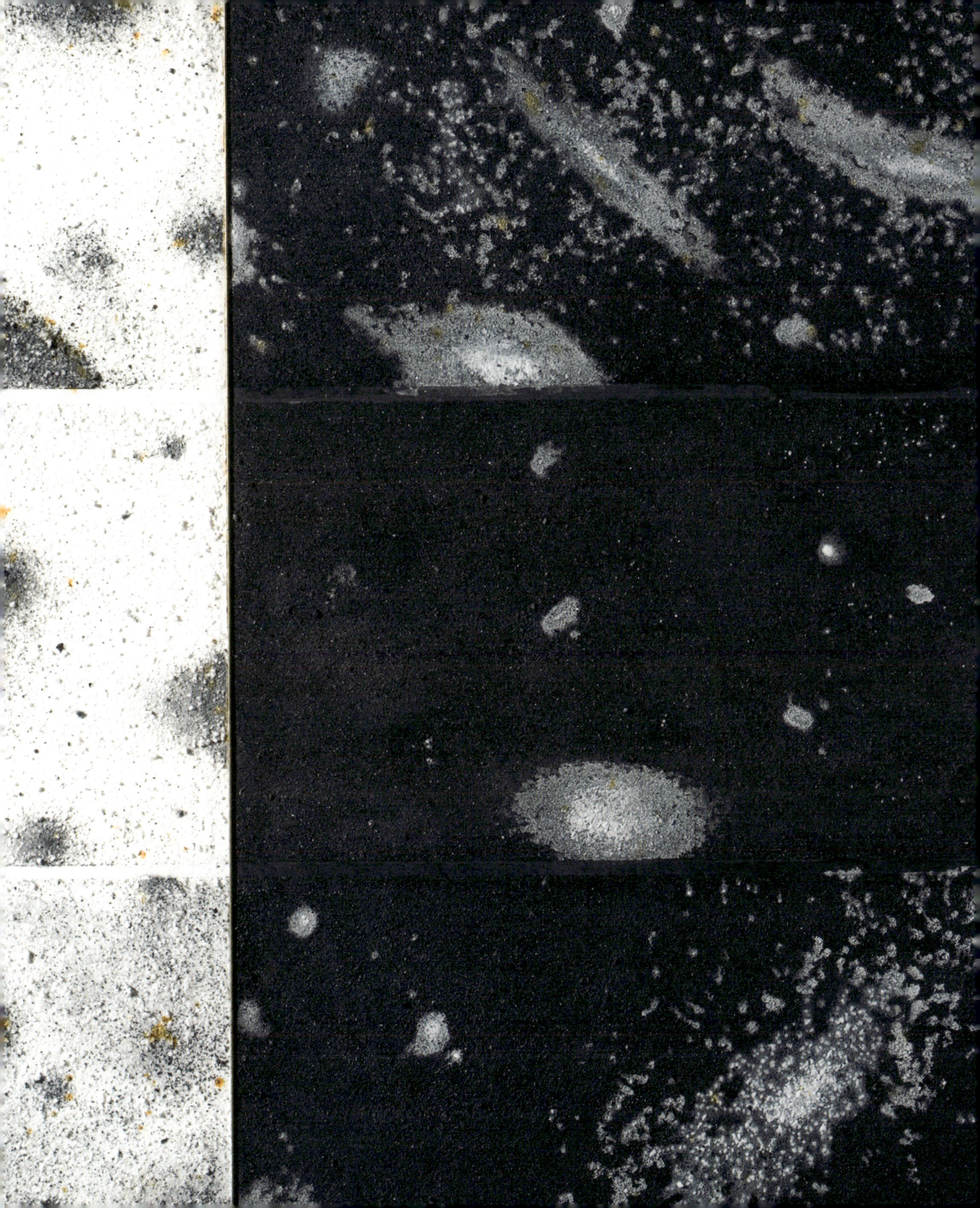

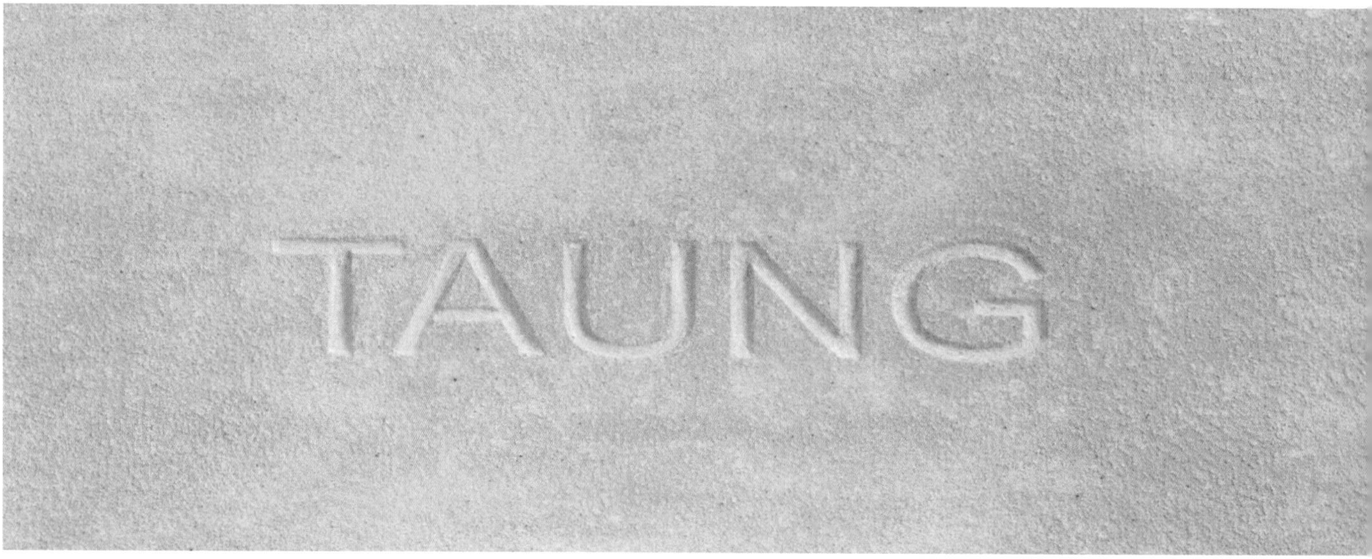

Karel Nel, *Taung/Piltdown*, site-specific dust/Fuller's earth (fake theatrical dust), 35 x 150 cm each (detail), 2011.

the universe itself. And it is precisely through his use of an alternative visual and metaphorical modality that his work is a contribution to knowledge-making – synthesising, in a different form, the questions prompted by scientific research and writing.

Nel's work is a meditation on the integration of the conceptual and the physical. His focus on the relationship between material objects, or matter, and the significance afforded them by humans brings to mind Ratele's observations on what can be said about skulls, or bones generally, and his insight that 'without stories, skulls are dead'.[13] Seemingly, it is story, or the construction of explanation around absent information that grounds the significance of bones,

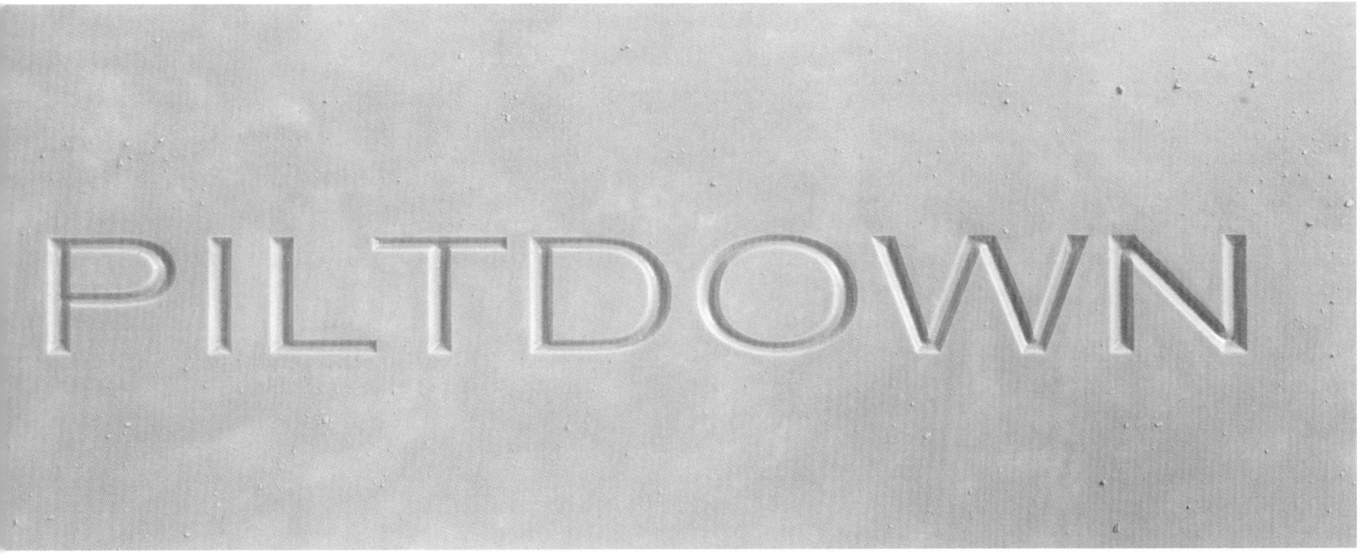

or intangible DNA evidence. Reading DNA sequences is linked to a narrative construction of individual and collective history. In Soodyall's comment, 'the body, through its DNA, constitutes an archive, with a narrative of our prehistory and evolutionary past'.[14]

In Chapter 4, Ratele considers the concurrent roles of invention, inventiveness, science and an imagination that always runs through accounts about lives (and bones), and how science and art themselves are part of those accounts. He considers Brenner's multitude of watercolour paintings, presented for the first time as a single body of work. They are daily meditations made from a close observation of and communion with the two human skulls and a cast of the

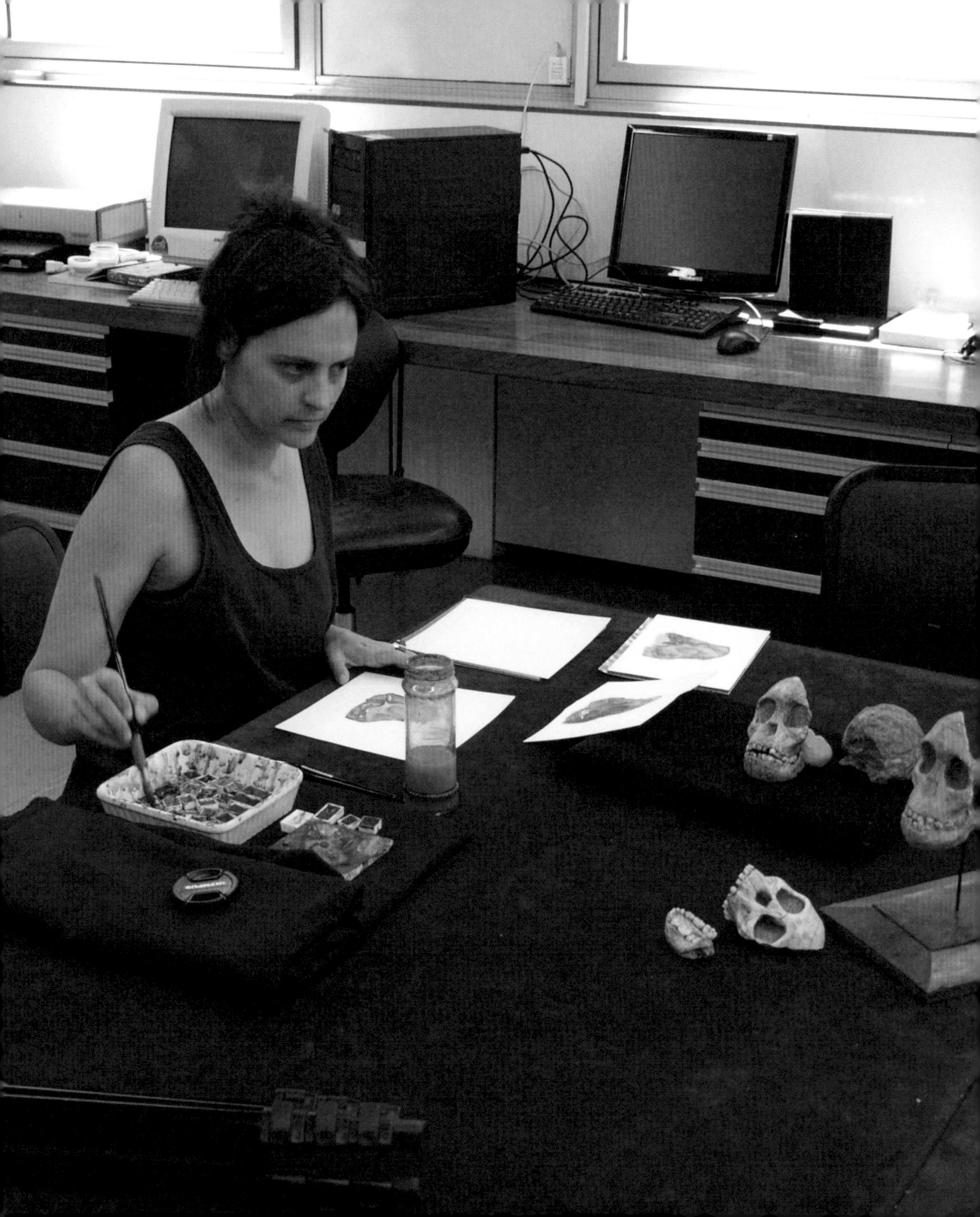

Taung fossil that she has in her studio. She also presents work made from direct observation of the Taung fossil at the Wits Medical School. Brenner's work in the field of portraiture turned a few years ago to a close examining of the internal structure of the head – not looking at the façade, but working to understand the inner architecture. This has prompted thought on what it is to be human and on the combined forces of the natural and the experiential or social, which make us the people we are. In many ways, her emotional and moody representations of skulls weave life, or presence, around absence. Each image is inevitably an intersection of self and object, of present and past; each one a specific observation combined with interpretation, simultaneously a focus and a projection. Each so different from the others, the paintings resulting from her daily looking at the same specimens yield a myriad of differences, rather than sameness. They reflect her interest in the stubbornly partial or fragmented ways in which we know others and ourselves. It is this frustration of not fully 'knowing' and of the impossibility of knowing that has been the point of connection with Ratele's meditations on truth and evidence, and on the cultural and scientific significance of bones.

Burroughs presents three works of creative non-fiction, one for each of the three artists represented in *Life of bone*. Her essays offer intimate insights into the ways artists think and work, the everyday realities of life and living that impact on the choices and decisions artists make. Burroughs weaves biographical accounts about the three artists and in so doing she asserts the significance of the personal crises, passions and impulses that drive practice. Her reflections are imaginatively reconstructed fragments of the lives of the three artists and bring to the fore a completely different attitude to the analysis and interpretation of art and art-making. While Burroughs unpacks and unpicks the construction of knowledge in terms of the artists' ways, her essays allude simultaneously to the ways of scientists.

Her intuitive yet intellectual approach to writing about the lives and work of the artists draws together past experience and present insight into a seamless account. She understands how 'feelings, ideas, emotions, loss and pleasure are the loam that nurture the next painting, and the next'. It is a way of working

Joni Brenner working at the Medical School in the Phillip Tobias Fossil Primate and Hominid Laboratory, 2010. Photograph by Bernhard Zipfel.

that resonates powerfully with anthropologist Tim Ingold's understanding of storylines and plots:

> I have suggested that drawing a line on a sketch map is much like telling a story. Indeed, the two commonly proceed in tandem as complementary strands of one and the same performance. Thus the storyline goes *along*, as does the line on the map. The things of which the story tells, let us say, do not so much exist as occur: each is a moment of ongoing activity. These things, in a word, are not objects but topics. Lying at the confluence of actions and responses, every topic is identified by its relations to the things that paved the way for it, that presently concur with it and that follow it into the world. Here the meaning of the 'relation' has to be understood quite literally, not as a connection between pre located entities but as a path traced through the terrain of lived experience. Far from connecting points in a network, every relation is one line in a meshwork of interwoven trails. To tell a story, then, is to *relate*, in narrative, the occurrences of the past, retracing a path through the world that others, recursively picking up the threads of past lives, can follow in the process of spinning out their own. But rather as in looping or knitting, the thread being spun now and the thread picked up from the past are both from the same yarn. There is no point at which the story ends and life begins.[15]

The elements of the exhibition

Central to the *Life of bone* exhibition is the display of the three parts that make up the small Taung fossilised skull: the incomplete skullbone, the jaw with its neat milk teeth and the endocranial cast, which Zipfel rightly describes as beautiful. Also on display is the rare Border Cave 1 specimen, which is a very early modern human skull, also fossilised, and a contemporary chimpanzee skull. An articulated cast of the Taung fossil is also on display, showing how the three pieces fit together. The skulls encapsulate a trajectory of time and evolution and their relationship to each other provokes a great deal of thought. The development of

Joni Brenner, Maquette for installation of *Wall of skulls*, composite photographs, 26 x 64 cm (detail), 2011.

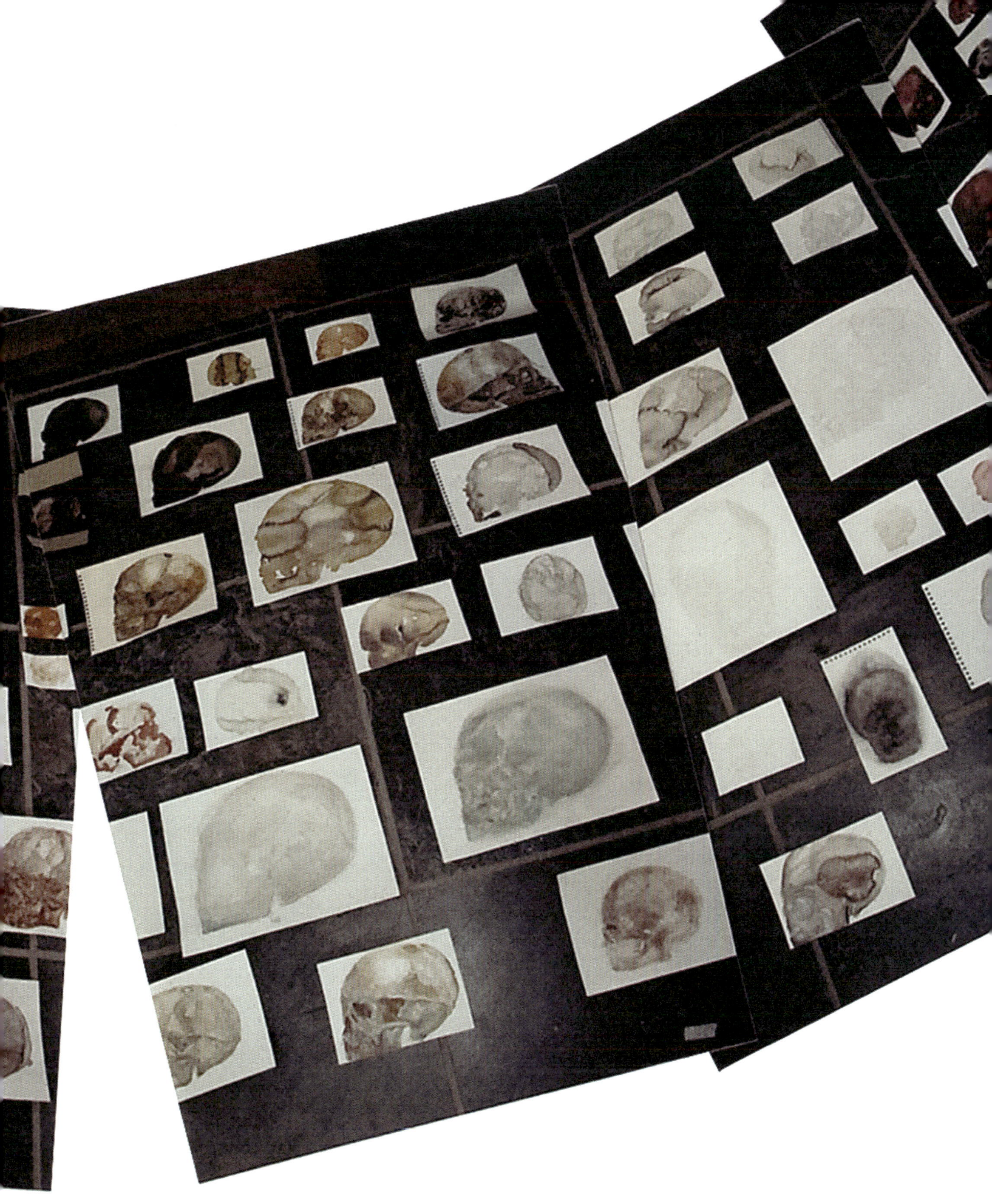

scientific thought proceeds through a range of investigative practices including hypothesis, experiment, comparative study and description.

On the walls surrounding the cabinets of skulls are artworks made by the three artists: Brenner, Marx and Nel. Their works engage with the evolutionary path embodied by the presence of the skulls, and, like a visual metaphor for the continuum of scientific interrogations of fossils and their relationship to our own sense of location, the artworks – in proximity to the 'evidence' – give rise to their own kind of interrogation. The artworks probe the spiritual or emotional links between ancient hominid ancestors and modern human beings and offer a different perspective. Indeed, probing these links prompts thought about consciousness itself, what the level of hominid consciousness was and how, perhaps, when consciousness becomes expressed and lingual, it takes on another dimension: recorded in memory and beyond it, an autobiographical sense of oneself and of one's own history becomes possible.

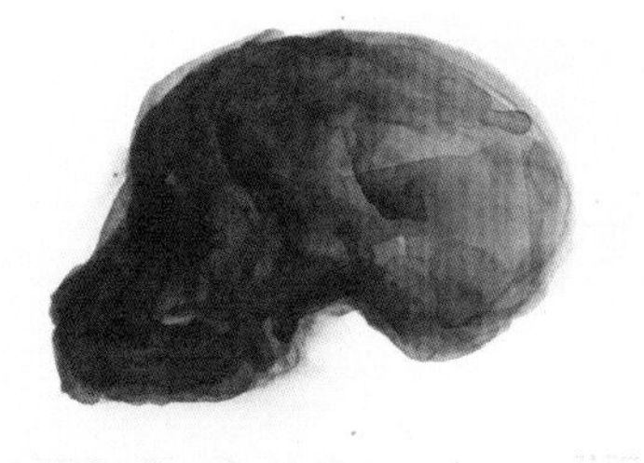

Joni Brenner, *Taung series*, watercolour on paper, 18 x 25.5 cm (detail left), 2009.

The human capacity for self-reflexivity creates the space for thought expressed in a variety of discourses that we have somehow tended to separate from each other. Although the artistic and scientific disciplines usually communicate in different dialects, when juxtaposed, as Stephen Jay Gould suggests, they reflect strikingly upon and enhance one another, producing a hybrid language richer than either could command on its own.[16]

Art meets science

All of the essays in this book reflect on the ways in which artists and scientists do their work, and on the similarities and differences in their approaches. In our attempts to demystify the processes of art and science, there is a focus in the essays on doing: on learning and thinking through doing. The development of scientific certainty – even if that certainty is always only temporary – happens through repetitive testing. Laboratory work is a repeated meditative form of doing that ensures proper quality control, especially in a diagnostic environment. Such iterative checking and cross-checking ensures that the research scientists do is reliable and reproducible. This kind of hands-on testing is the solid ground from which more intuitive and imaginative investigations can be launched. Learning through doing, much like Brenner's daily skull work, or any sustained artistic practice, may be meditative and soothing, but, driven as it is by a seeking impulse, is not idle.

The contributions in *Life of bone* consider the ways in which artworks add to knowledge, but they also explore how artworks themselves can exist as residues of knowledge-making. The Swiss-French artist, Alberto Giacometti, is interesting in this regard. His sculptures are sites of enquiry, struggle, trial and error. They are surfaces on and through which he was testing ideas, learning and understanding through doing. His biographer, James Lord, who also sat for Giacometti, wrote the following:

> ... it had also grown harder and harder for Alberto to see when a work was finished. Being finished meant that he could do no more with it. If he acknowledged that no more could be done, then, far from finishing a single painting or sculpture, he was admitting that none should have been started. This state of affairs, however, presented no problem to a man for whom the most important part of his work had long since become the part to be done the next day. He could see that part, because he saw that sculptures and paintings were never a likeness of what he saw. ... Whether [others] saw his work as completed or incomplete, to him it was all the same, *because works of art were not basically what he was looking for.* For him, a fragment was already immense, since a human arm could equal the extent of the Milky Way.[17] (italics added)

Giacometti's process of working can be likened to that of a scientist, driven by a passion, by a particular line of thought or by a stubborn problem. But, as Kemp points out, the kinds of knowledge produced by artists and scientists working often in the same kinds of ways are radically different: 'An image in art is a field for interpretation. Try as they may, artists cannot control the openness of the act of viewing. Scientists, however, try to cut down ambiguity in published work.'[18]

This is not to say that scientific explorations are not speculative, tentative and imaginative. They are. Good scientific research embraces the accidental and the incidental. It does not stick systematically to the formula of hypothesise, experiment, test, and conclude, though it will move constantly between the intuitively or imaginatively derived and the rigorously tested. All scientific knowledge is constructed slowly over time with new principles built on tested foundations of preceding knowledge, theories or principles, themselves having been subjected to rigorous testing by way of mathematical calculations or actual experiments that will have confirmed or refuted the new hypothesis. Prior knowledge strongly influences the establishment of new knowledge, and it may be that this conscious and deliberate aspect of the scientific process explains why the acceptance of new knowledge in a scientific community is generally painfully slow and shrouded in scepticism, with the new knowledge subjected to years of tests and interrogation. Nonetheless, while scientific outcomes are typically perceived as truth, they are often based on subjective hypotheses, and great scientific breakthroughs mostly take shape in combination with active imagination. A combination of exactness and playfulness defines the terrain.

John Dewey reminds us that 'every great advance in science has issued from a new audacity of imagination'.[19] Quantum theory, work on dark matter and theories about the origins of the universe provide ample evidence that much of science has become startlingly speculative.[20] Science too proceeds through interpreting, conjecturing, exploring, imagining – not only by way of explaining – and it poses many more questions than it answers. But the rigorous testing and slow establishment of conventionally accepted scientific knowledge is essential for the confirmation of the fabulous and the interesting; the rigour forms the background for the breakthrough.

So, both in science and in art, conventional and formulaic modes of research – if that is all there is – can be limiting and stultifying. Gerrit Olivier, an esteemed South African academic with a commitment to placing creative work on the same footing as more conventionally understood research, reflects on the pitfalls of a standard, formulaic approach to art-making. Olivier argues that creative research is necessarily different from standard academic research and considers

RIGHT: Karel Nel working in his Rivonia studio, Johannesburg. Photograph by John Hodgkiss, 2008.

that artistic work that abides by the more conventional scientific research methods runs the risk of being extremely boring:

> One puts forward a hypothesis ('I intend to play *The Goldberg Variations* in a new way to achieve a certain effect'), conducts research aimed at this outcome (analysing the score, reading about Bach, dissecting previous performances by Glenn Gould *et al.*), performs the work, reflects on the performance and researches its reception.[21]

Karel Nel, *Shift seam*, red Bengara pigment and black carboniferous dust, 51 x 51 cm, 2009.

He reflects that this would be 'putting a very complex and often unpredictable process within a framework that seems to deny its very open-endedness'.[22] Artworks, he goes on to say, are clearly 'not a straightforward, scientifically verifiable kind of knowledge. Instead, it is "knowledge" that appeals to more than our rational, analytic selves and is imbedded in the structure, texture and patterns of the work.[23] … Creative outputs are complex and public human expressions that contribute to the world in a variety of domains'.[24]

Similarly, Carl Jung acknowledges the importance for science to see its work as only one part of knowledge production:

> Science is the tool of the Western mind and with it more doors can be opened than with bare hands. It is part and parcel of our knowledge and obscures our insight only when it holds that the understanding given by it is the only kind there is.[25]

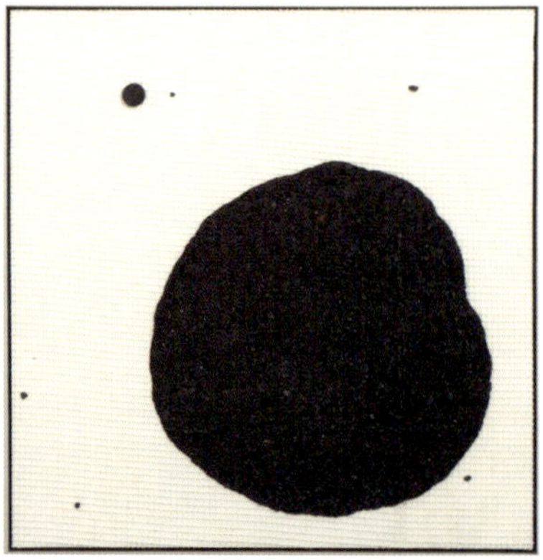

Karel Nel, *Stellar mask*, black carboniferous dust, white pigment, polythene grid, 51 x 51 cm, 2009.

In many ways, modern science is so abstract that the leaps of imagination required to understand the principles being established must make use of living metaphors (the Big Bang, black holes) almost as a precondition to facilitate understanding – both for scientists themselves and for the rest of us. Visual diagrams and metaphors are the mediating strategies, acting in much the same way as transformers do, representing abstract or vast quantities of data in ways that enable comprehension.

So, what can we learn from the dialogue emerging from the exhibition of the Taung child in conversation, as it were, with the artworks produced by Brenner, Marx and Nel? What are the connections between art and evolution? What can creative productions tell us about ourselves, in relation to scientific evidence or knowledge we may have about our origins? The philosopher, Dennis Dutton, suggests that:

> The evolution of *Homo sapiens* in the past million years is not just a history of how we came to have acute colour vision, a taste for sweets, and an upright gait. It is also a story of how we became a species obsessed with creating artistic experiences with which to amuse, shock, titillate, and enrapture ourselves, from children's games to the quartets of Beethoven, from firelit caves to the continuous worldwide glow of television screens.[26]

Dutton's line of thinking posits art-making as an instinct, as an evolutionary development, and perhaps such a proposition helps to form a tighter web of connecting lines between the skulls and the artworks on this exhibition.

In as much as the skulls themselves are traces of part of the story of origins, the maps and roots redeployed by Marx, Brenner's scores of emotive watercolour meditations on being, or the dust sampled by Nel as a trace of time and event, serve to imbue these objects from the past with contemporary significance.

Dutton writes that 'mitochondrial-DNA and Y-chromosome studies tell us facts about genetic histories we never would have dreamed of knowing in the past'[27] and it is true, we know much more than any other generation has known about our past, and about our long historical past.

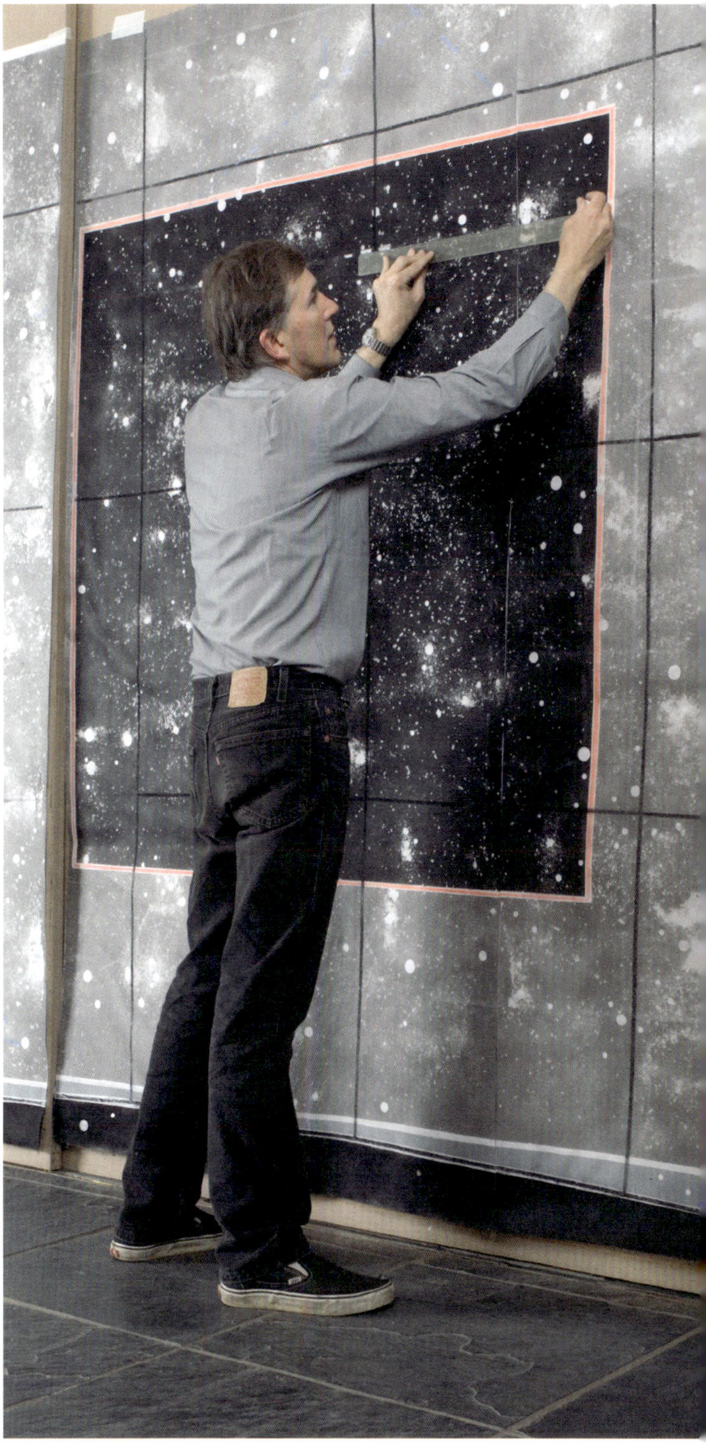

Why has the impulse to explore through artistic modalities survived, and with such sustained viewer interest? Is making art, as Dutton suggests, part of our genetic make-up? His assertion, or hypothesis, creates the next round of questions and demonstrates that the more we know, the more we realise there is to know.

The visual and textual conversations represented in *Life of bone* reflect on the making of art and the making of science. They consider the role of the imaginative in the progression of knowledge, and speak of the many ways in which there are gaps in knowledge. Knowledge of these gaps leads to 'worrying at the bone', the very process that resolves anomalies, finds new answers and elicits novel questions.

Notes

1 Kemp, M. 2010. "A Second Renaissance" in *New Scientist*. May 8, p. 44.

2 Eliot, T.S. 1971. "Tradition and the Individual Talent" in *Critical Theory Since Plato.* Adams, H (ed). New York: Harcourt Brace Jovanovich. p. 762.

3 Baxandall, M. 1985. *Patterns of Intention: On the Historical Explanation of Pictures*. New Haven and London: Yale University Press. pp. 58,59.

4 Bal, M. 1999. *Quoting Caravaggio: Contemporary Art: Preposterous History*. Chicago: University of Chicago Press.

5 Bryson, N. 2003. "Bacon's dialogues with the past" in *Francis Bacon and the Tradition of Art*. Milan: Skira. p. 43.

6 Hallam, E. 2010. "Articulating bones: an epilogue" in *Journal of Material Culture*. 15(4), p. 465.

7 Lewin, R. 1987. *Bones of contention*. Chicago: University of Chicago Press.

8 Krmpotich, C., Fontein, J. and Harries, J. (eds). 2010. "The substance of bones: the emotive materiality and affective presence of human remains" in *Journal of Material Culture*. Special Edition 15(4), pp. 371–384.

9 These comic-strip brochures entitled "Routes to Roots" are a product of the MRC/NHLS/Wits Human Genomic Diversity and Disease Research Unit and are distributed to communities that participate in Soodyall's fieldwork research undertaken as part of the human genome mapping project.

10 Kemp. 'A Second Renaissance'. p. 44.

11 Nel, K. 2009. "Disrupted knowledge" in *Penelope and the Cosmos*. Johannesburg: Circa on Jellicoe. p. 12.

12 Johanson, D. and Edgar, B. 1996. *From Lucy to Language*. London: Weidenfeld and Nicolson. p. 21.

13 Ratele, K. 2009, July 24. Email to Joni Brenner.

14 Hamilton, C. *et al*. (eds). 2002. *Refiguring the archive*. Cape Town: David Phillip Publishers. p. 180.

15 Ingold, T. 2007. *Lines: a brief history*. New York: Routledge. p. 90.

16 Gould, S.J. and Purcell, R. 2000. *Crossing Over: Where Art and Science Meet*. New York: Three Rivers Press. (quote from front sleeve).

17 Lord, J. 1983. *Giacometti, A Biography*. New York: Farrar, Straus, Giroux. p. 399.

18 Kemp, M. 2010. 'A Second Renaissance' in New Scientist. May 8, p. 44

19 Dewey, J. 1929. *The Quest for Certainty: A Study of the Relation of Knowledge and Action*. New York: Minton, Balch & Company. p. 310.

20 Olivier, G. 2010. "Formal recognition for creative work: some critical reflections" in *On Making: Integrating Approaches to Practice-Led Research in Art and Design*. Farber, L. (ed). Johannesburg: The Research Centre, *Visual Identities in Art and Design*, University of Johannesburg. p. 81.

21 ibid. p. 86.

22 ibid. p. 86.

23 ibid. p. 83.

24 ibid. p. 86.

25 Jung, C. and Wilhelm, R. 1931. *The Secret of the Golden Flower*. London: Kegan Paul, Trench, Trubner. p. 78.

26 Dutton, D. 2009. *The Art Instinct: Beauty, Pleasure, and Human Evolution*. New York, Berlin, London: Bloomsbury Press. p. 3.

27 ibid. p. 247.

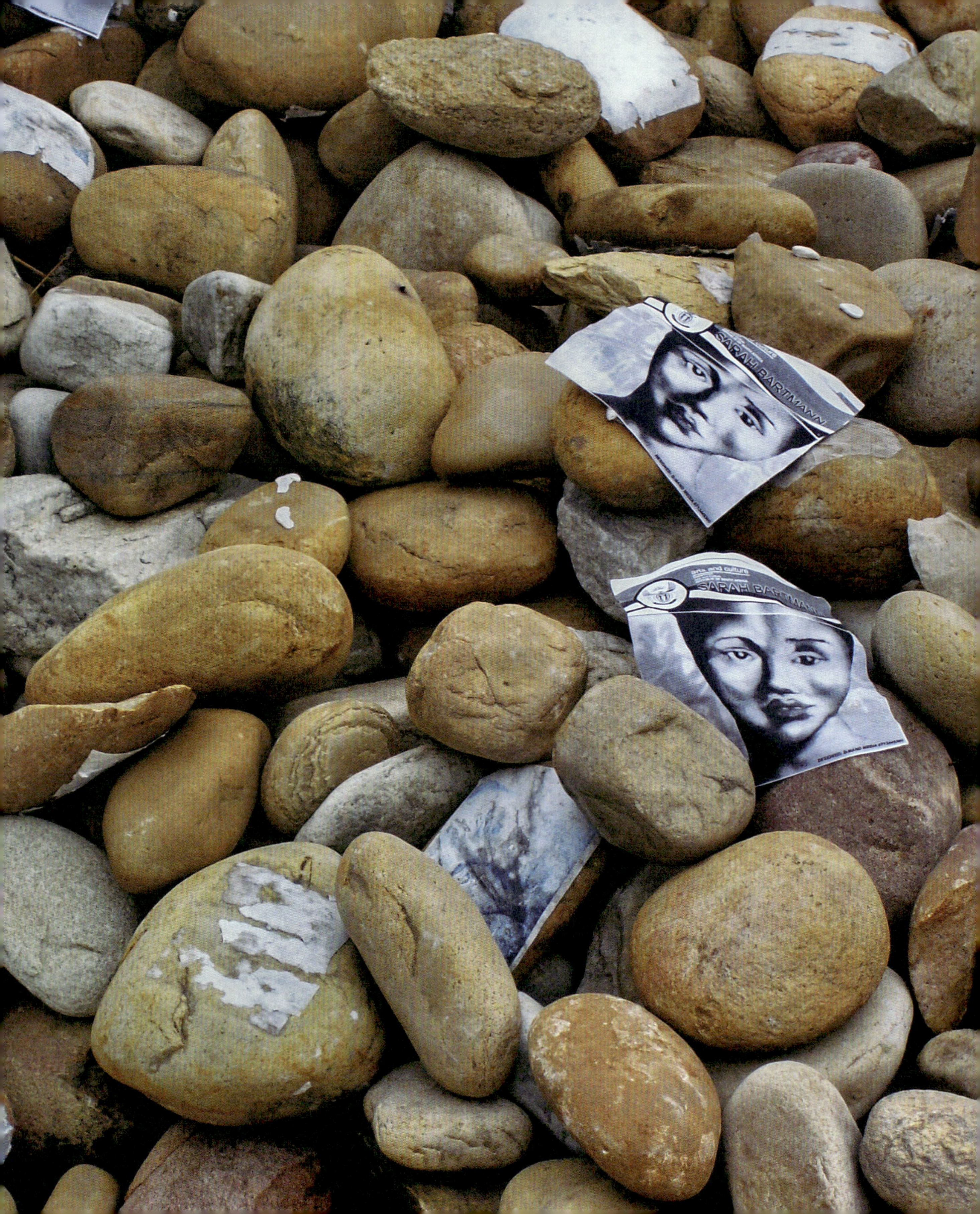
SARAH BARTMANN
arts and culture
SARAH BARTMANN

Chapter 2

History, ancestry and genes

Himla Soodyall

Friday, August 9, 2002 – Hankey, Eastern Cape. Amidst the sounds of singing women, the smell of strong incense, burning Khoigoed and the gaze of several members of Khoisan cultural groups, I broke the seal of one of the jars that contained the remains of the brain tissue of Sarah Bartmann, which was dissected and preserved after her death in 1816[1]. I handed the remains to a representative of the Khoisan group. A pungent smell of solvent, perhaps formaldehyde, mixed with alcohol filled my nostrils. Tears rolled down my cheeks – either a reaction to the sharp smell or the overwhelming emotion I felt from conducting the task I was charged with on behalf of the Sarah Bartmann Reference Group.[2] I felt a strong urge to throw up. I started coughing again – the smoke and the smells were getting to me. Knowing that the next task was to break the seal of the second jar, the one carrying Bartmann's genital tissue, I leaned over to reach for the jar. The singing and the crying intensified. The jar was a bit further away, so I had to stretch over the buckets to reach for it. My gloves were now wet from the contents of the first jar, and I thought it was going to slip through my fingers. Someone helped me, and together we managed to get the jar open and it was with relief that I handed the contents over and heard the glass jar crash into the bucket below. I looked across and there, in a crate, lay the skeletal remains of Bartmann, respectfully packed in foam padding in the correct anatomical position, but the Khoisan

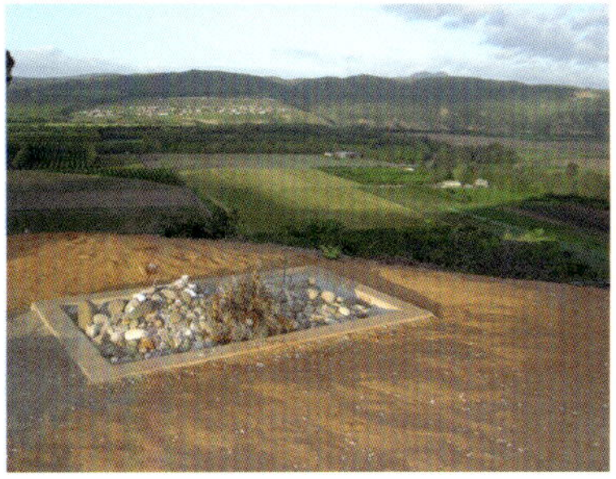

Sarah Bartmann grave, Hankey.
Photograph by John Wait, 2002.

LEFT: Sarah Bartmann grave, Hankey.
Photograph by Deborah Lepojevic. 2007.

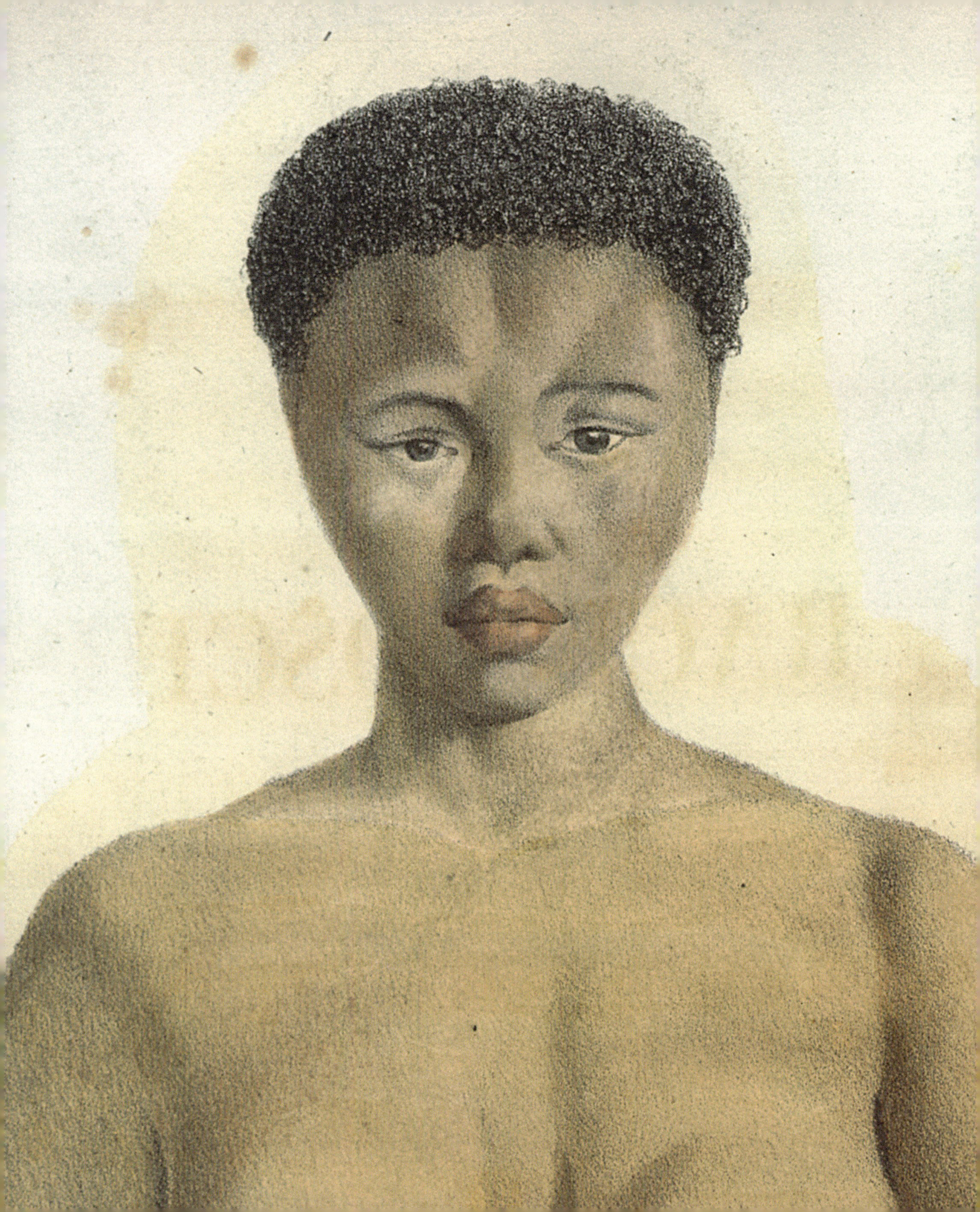

representatives lifted the bones from the crate and wrapped them snugly in animal skin for the interment process.

'Femme de race Bochismann' (detail) after de Wailly, Geoffrey-Saint-Hilaire and Frédéric Cuvier, Coloured lithograph, 29 x 49 cm, 1824, courtesy The British Library.

The singing continued with the ritual of preparing her remains for burial. I could not believe how my life as a scientist had now intersected in a very special way with an icon of South African history. I was standing at the burial site and watching the interment ceremony with dignitaries including former president Thabo Mbeki, other representatives of government, academics, intellectuals, cultural workers, community leaders, the Reference Group, the media, and members of the Hankey and Kouga regions, all of us joined together to restore dignity to Bartmann's life. Hearing the poem written for Bartmann by Diana Ferrus,[3] brought life to the bones:

I've come to take you home –
home, remember the veld?
the lush green grass beneath the big oak trees
the air is cool there and the sun does not burn.
I have made your bed at the foot of the hill,
your blankets are covered in buchu and mint,
the proteas stand in yellow and white
and the water in the stream chuckle sing-songs
as it hobbles along over little stones.

I have come to wrench you away –
away from the poking eyes
of the man-made monster
who lives in the dark
with his clutches of imperialism
who dissects your body bit by bit
who likens your soul to that of Satan
and declares himself the ultimate god!

'Sartjee, the Hottentot Venus, Now Exhibiting in London, Drawn From Life', hand-coloured line engraving, 23 x 36 cm, 1810, courtesy City of Westminster Archives Centre.

I have come to soothe your heavy heart
I offer my bosom to your weary soul
I will cover your face with the palms of my hands
I will run my lips over lines in your neck
I will feast my eyes on the beauty of you
and I will sing for you
for I have come to bring you peace.

I have come to take you home
where the ancient mountains shout your name.
I have made your bed at the foot of the hill,
your blankets are covered in buchu and mint,
the proteas stand in yellow and white
I have come to take you home
where I will sing for you
for you have brought me peace.

People of all cultural backgrounds, representing the South African nation, were assembled to achieve a common purpose – remembering and honouring Sarah Bartmann. In doing so, we also had to understand our South African history and the origins and diversity of all people who live here. More importantly, the occasion reminded us that people suffer discrimination, marginalisation and human rights violations, and by respecting Bartmann's remains, we were also here to ensure that such gross violations of human rights do not happen again.

Looking at skeletal remains

Since I was raised a Hindu, I am familiar with the custom of cremation, rather than burial, following the death of a family member. After the funeral service and cremation, the only bond or connection with the deceased individual is through memories of how our lives intersected. There is no memorial or grave to visit. Thus,

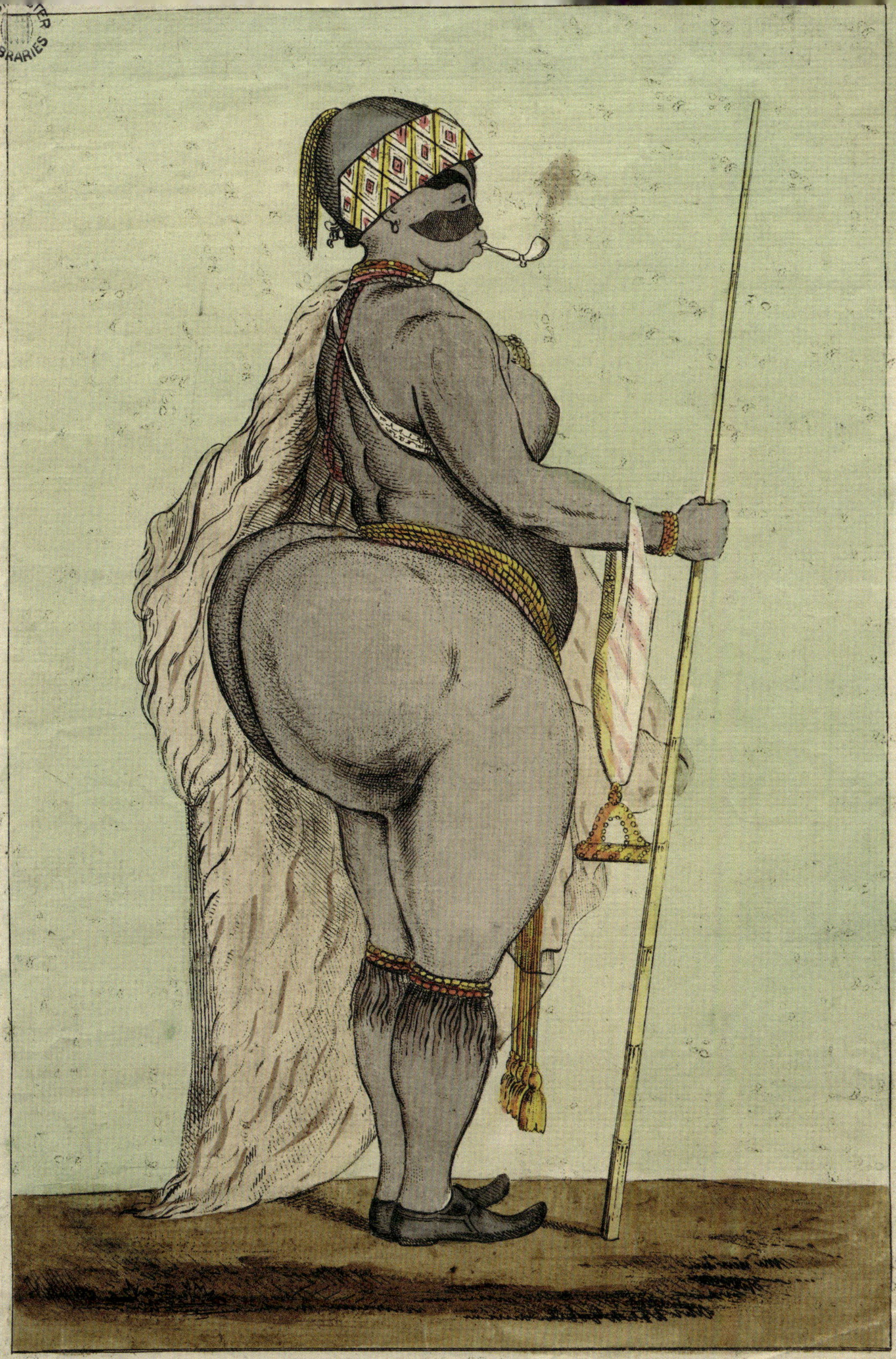

SARTLEE, THE HOTTENTOT VENUS.

Now Exhibiting in London.

Drawn from Life

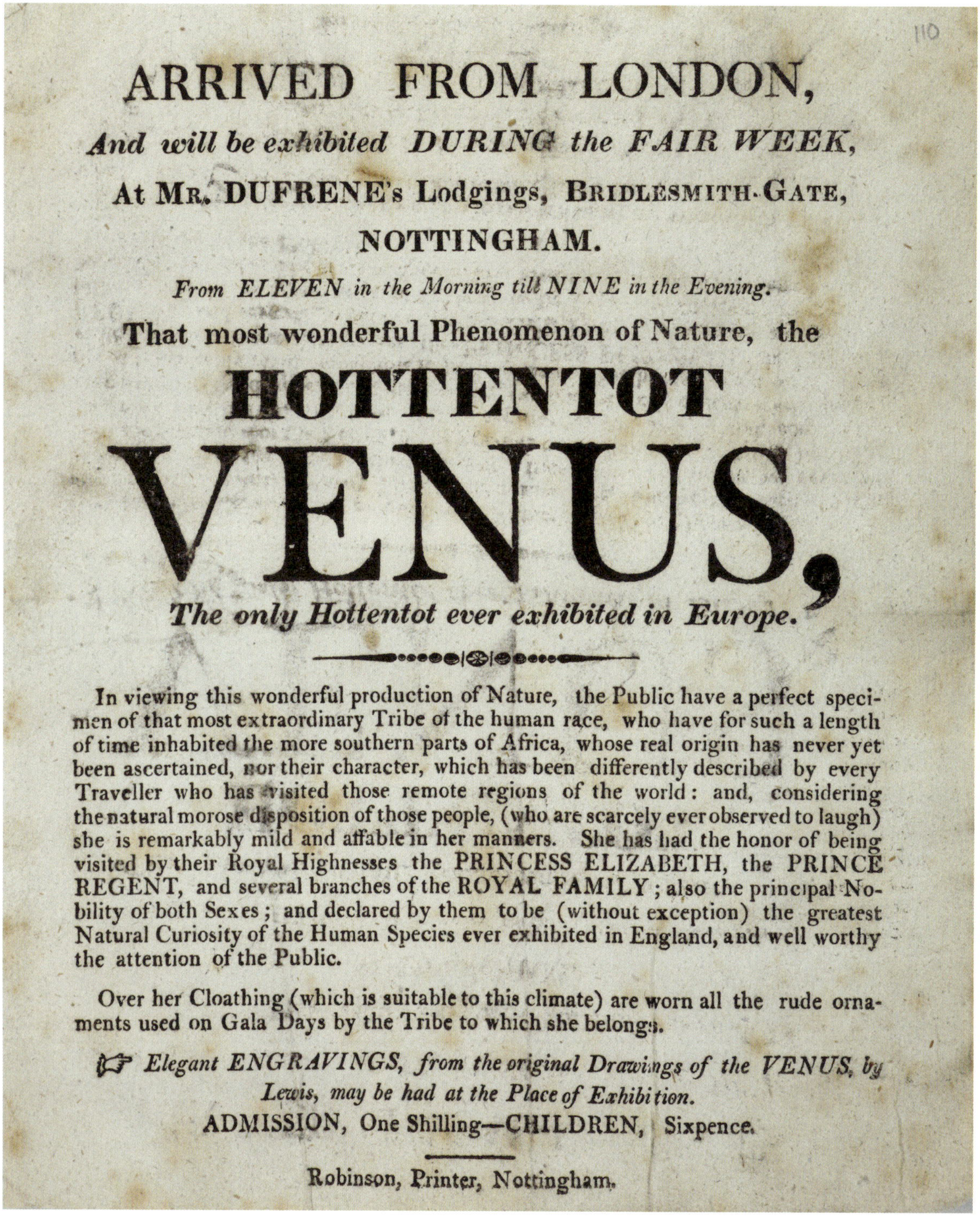

ARRIVED FROM LONDON,

And will be exhibited ***DURING*** *the* ***FAIR WEEK,***

At MR. DUFRENE's Lodgings, BRIDLESMITH-GATE,

NOTTINGHAM.

From ELEVEN in the Morning till NINE in the Evening.

That most wonderful Phenomenon of Nature, the

HOTTENTOT

VENUS,

The only Hottentot ever exhibited in Europe.

In viewing this wonderful production of Nature, the Public have a perfect specimen of that most extraordinary Tribe of the human race, who have for such a length of time inhabited the more southern parts of Africa, whose real origin has never yet been ascertained, nor their character, which has been differently described by every Traveller who has visited those remote regions of the world: and, considering the natural morose disposition of those people, (who are scarcely ever observed to laugh) she is remarkably mild and affable in her manners. She has had the honor of being visited by their Royal Highnesses the PRINCESS ELIZABETH, the PRINCE REGENT, and several branches of the ROYAL FAMILY; also the principal Nobility of both Sexes; and declared by them to be (without exception) the greatest Natural Curiosity of the Human Species ever exhibited in England, and well worthy the attention of the Public.

Over her Cloathing (which is suitable to this climate) are worn all the rude ornaments used on Gala Days by the Tribe to which she belongs.

☞ *Elegant ENGRAVINGS, from the original Drawings of the VENUS, by Lewis, may be had at the Place of Exhibition.*

ADMISSION, One Shilling—CHILDREN, Sixpence.

Robinson, Printer, Nottingham.

the experience of being in the immediate vicinity of skeletal remains aroused an intense uneasiness in me, and reminded me of the first time I had to work on a sample of foetal tissue where my responsibility was to confirm a diagnosis for an inherited disease.

Poster announcing the appearance of Sarah Baartman, Robinson, printer, Nottingham, 22 x 19 cm, ca.1811, courtesy The British Library.

Yet, I am fascinated by how the discovery of hominid fossils piques our scientific curiosity and furthers our knowledge. In some instances, accidental discoveries like that of the Taung child, or planned excavations such as the one at Border Cave, unearth specimens dating back thousands or even millions of years. Through these research efforts, scientists have been able to posit, for example, that Neandertals were the first hominids to bury the dead intentionally, doing so in shallow graves along with stone tools and animal bones.[4]

When Stephen Jay Gould visited the Musée de l'Homme in Paris, the specificity of viewing Bartmann's remains, not to mention Descartes' skull and the brain of Broca, among the preserved brains of other named, white male scientists,[5] struck him with such personal force that he wrote and published an essay entitled 'The Hottentot Venus'. This essay and former president Nelson Mandela's personal appeal for the return of Bartmann's remains to her country were instrumental in persuading the French to repatriate the remains.

It is sobering to consider that Bartmann's skeleton was exhibited publically without scruple for many years, then stored away in the Musée de l'Homme before finally making its journey back home for a dignified burial. Our experience with skeletal remains thus also differs in relation to how far back in time they date. Identifiable remains such as Bartmann's affect us differently to much older and fossilised remains where a level of detachment seems possible.

Gerhard Marx is an artist whose work has engaged with the portrayal of human remains as well as with people close to death. Writing of his own experiences with skulls and skeletons, he observes:

> Looking at the skeleton has been a source of ambiguous curiosity in my work. This curiosity does not lie in the object or the image, but lies in the fact that the skull or skeleton is difficult or even impossible to look at, almost impossible to see. On the one hand, one cannot look at these objects without the consistent,

nagging interruption of the imagination. The imagination flourishes with narrative embellishments, anthropomorphic or empathetic constructions and fictional projections, which veil the object with imagined histories. On the other hand, the same holds true for reason: logic desperately proliferates explanations, grapples with time frames, practicalities and forensic explanations. The act of looking at the skull (or skeleton) sends both imagination and reason into a frenzied and conflicting, irreconcilable state: the two attempt to marry imaginings with theories, but fail to find satisfactory conclusions.

Human remains, particularly bone, are an object-type that I think of as self-effacing. These objects (like maps, photos, fossils) operate in a totally indexical manner. This category of object always unfailingly points away from itself, towards an excess, towards an exteriority or event that has taken place elsewhere, towards a life that was. The insistence with which these objects point away from themselves obsessively negates their own presence, to a degree of near invisibility, camouflaged as they are, in allusion.

Of course, the conscious body finds the vision of its own organism's disorganisation unbearable. The functioning totality, the organism built through the organisation of organs, resists the idea of itself as dissipated. This identification may be precisely what drives that primary human impulse: the burial of the dead. When the body is faced with a fragmented version of itself (as skull, skeleton or tissue), the living body buries it in the rich soil of myth, scientific explanation, religious rumination or philosophical contemplation. The very act of looking at the skull (or skeleton) dresses the bone with phantom, storied flesh.

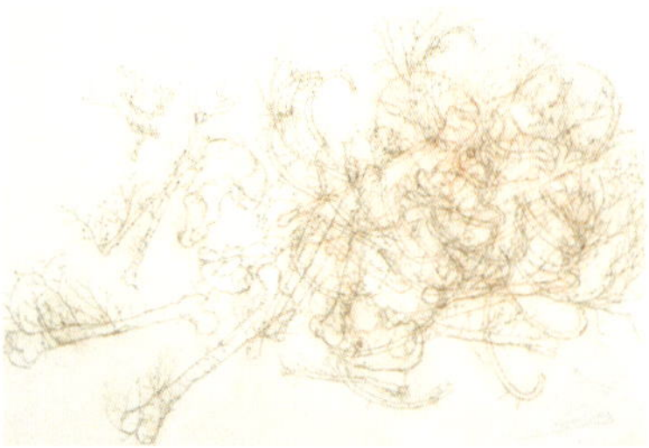

Gerhard Marx, *Cumulus II*, plant material, acrylic paint and glue on cotton paper, 153 x 103 cm (detail right), 2011.

Marx's observations on skeletons help us to understand how the burial of Bartmann recontextualises the use of her remains from that of 'scientific explanation' of difference, into that of political myth-making. Over and above this contemporary use, however, there is also the very genuine and human desire to lay to rest a life and a body so badly misused.

Georges Bataille[6] asserts that humans are distinguished from animals in our knowledge of our death. Like Marx, Posel and Gupta wonder whether it is possible that humans' knowledge of death and dying ties into our imminent repugnance

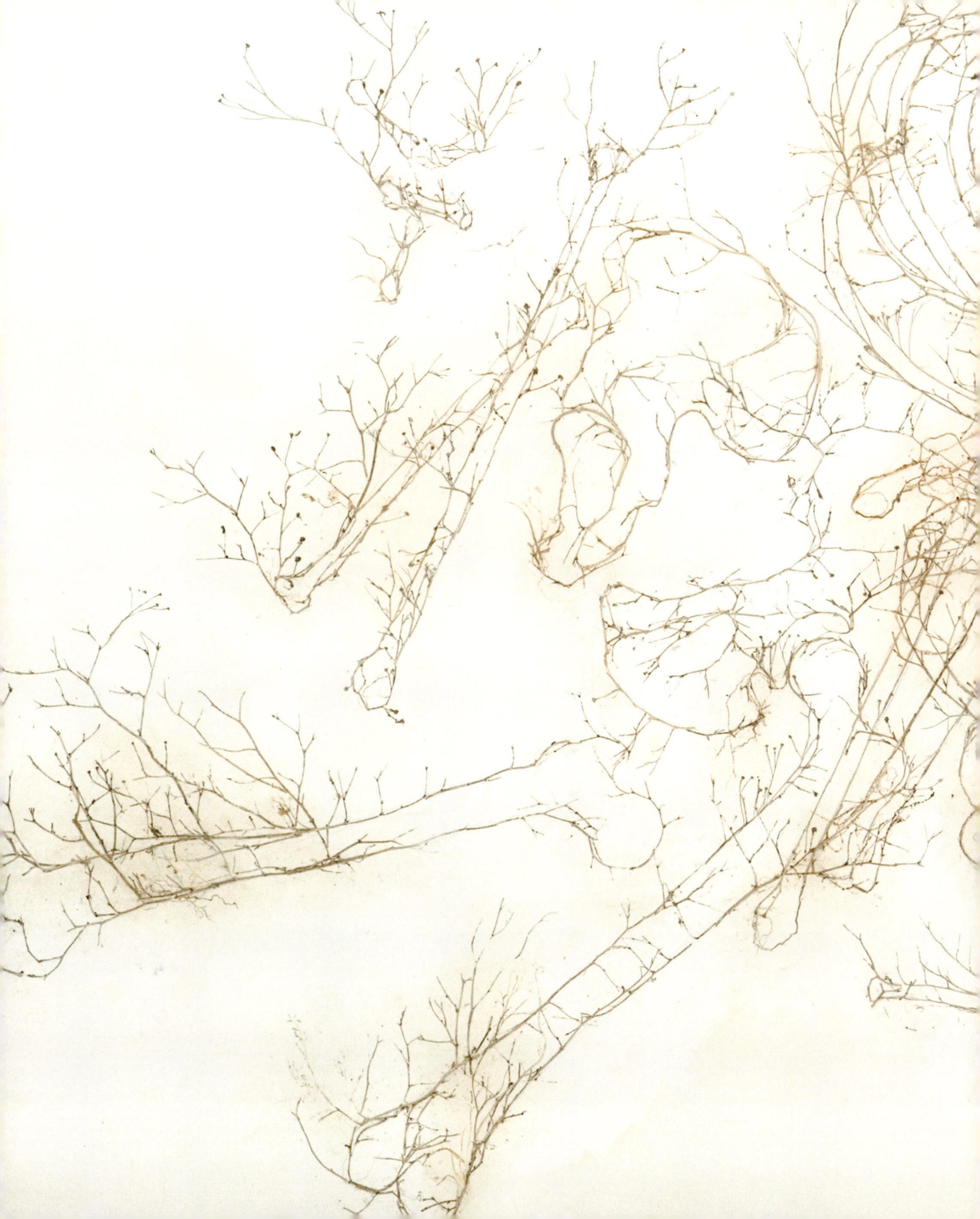

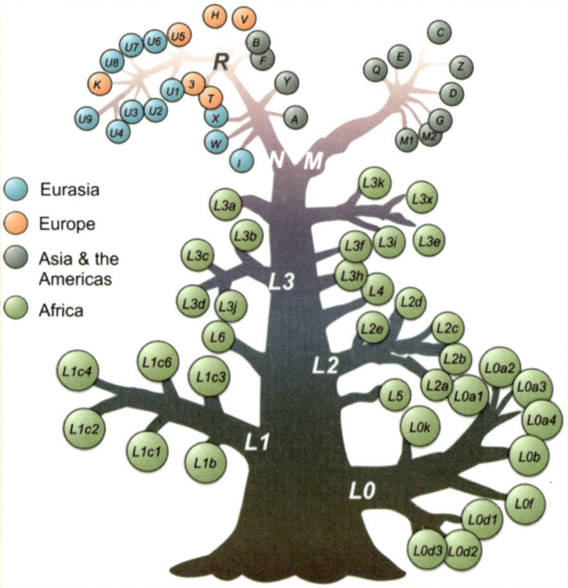

In the tree featured above, mtDNA found in living people would be represented as leaves which would be anchored via their twigs to small branches, which eventually merge into bigger branches until all branches connect to the trunk. Each circle on this tree represents a mtDNA branch (or haplogroup). The colours show the most likely geographic region of origin of the mtDNA branch. L0 is the deepest branch on the tree, and L0d is the branch that harbours the majority of the mtDNA lineages found among the Khoi and San. Over time, as humans migrated out of Africa to populate the rest of the world, they took with them a subset of the divergent mtDNA lineages found in Africa, which eventually mutated or changed to produce the various lineages found in living people outside of Africa. At the same time, those ancestors who remained in Africa continued to evolve newer lineages. As people migrated and settled throughout the continent, their contact with other groups contributed to gene exchange between groups thereby contributing to shaping the gene pool found in living people.

In the past 20 years or so, researchers have studied several populations throughout the world and have mapped the global patterns of mtDNA variation. There is reasonable concordance between one's geographic region of origin and the mtDNA lineages found in that region.

In addition to mtDNA, Y-chromosome DNA offers an equivalent tool to trace paternal heritage (father, father's father, great grandfather, etc) in males. Y-chromosome patterns of variation are also highly structured by geographic region. Also, specific Y-chromosome changes or mutations have been identified that contribute to the branching pattern of the Y-chromosome tree.

or disgust for death and dead bodies as well as our human impulse or compulsion to restore dignity at the moment that a body shifts to becoming a corpse.[7]

History, genes and trees

Humans have pondered their origins for as long as they have existed. This wondering is reflected in the many myths and creation stories. We need only think about the Judeo-Christian Garden of Eden, for example. Indeed, such stories of origin seem to be a nearly universal feature of human cultures. Nowadays, we reconstruct human history using a number of different methods. In the absence of written records, scholars have made use of information from disciplines as diverse as linguistics, archaeology, physical anthropology, cultural anthropology, history and palaeoanthropology to reconstruct our prehistory. The most direct account of our past is inferred from the fossil record. Skeletal remains, like the Taung skull, have been instrumental in establishing the evolution of human ancestors in Africa, and they have also provided important information about the evolution of modern *Homo sapiens*.

We all identify with the family unit and our family tree: siblings, parents, grandparents, great-grandparents and so forth. Even without really understanding the complexities of biological inheritance, we are quick to recognise that certain physical traits (for example, hair colour, nose shape, height) as well as behavioural traits (like temperament, voice, temper) run in the family. How often have we heard people say 'you have your mother's smile' or 'you have a temper like your grandpa'? Identifying with family – kinship – and paying respect to our ancestors is part of our cultural evolution. Solomon Plaatje, the esteemed South African intellectual, journalist, linguist, politician, translator and writer, was particularly proud of his Barolong ancestry. He reconstructed his genealogical history, believing that he was the first in his family to put memory to paper. He traced his paternal ancestry to King Morolong who is believed to have lived during the 12th or 13th century. He also traced his maternal ancestry to Tau, the founder of the four royal branches of the Barolong. Plaatje deduced from the genealogical data that his father and mother shared a common ancestry but 27 degrees apart.[8] Mandela also acknowledges his ancestry in his autobiography, *The long walk to freedom*. He refers to his father, Gadla Henry Mphakanyiswa, as a chief by both blood and custom who belonged to the Thembu tribe.[9]

Unfortunately, few of us have access to good genealogical information, and even when present, genealogical information can only take us back relatively few generations. Genetic information on the other hand, the biochemical instructions that determine inherited traits, provide us with an indelible record of our evolutionary past. Thus, by studying DNA in living people, it is possible to reconstruct how specific regions of the human genome, which by virtue of their unique mode of inheritance, can be traced back to a common point in the past. For example, mitochondrial DNA (mtDNA), which is inherited exclusively from our mothers (mother, maternal grandmother, maternal great-grandmother, and so on), provides us with the opportunity to trace our maternal ancestry several thousands of years back. Both sons and daughters inherit their mothers' mtDNA, but only the daughters will pass their mtDNA to their offspring. Thus all mtDNA lineages found in

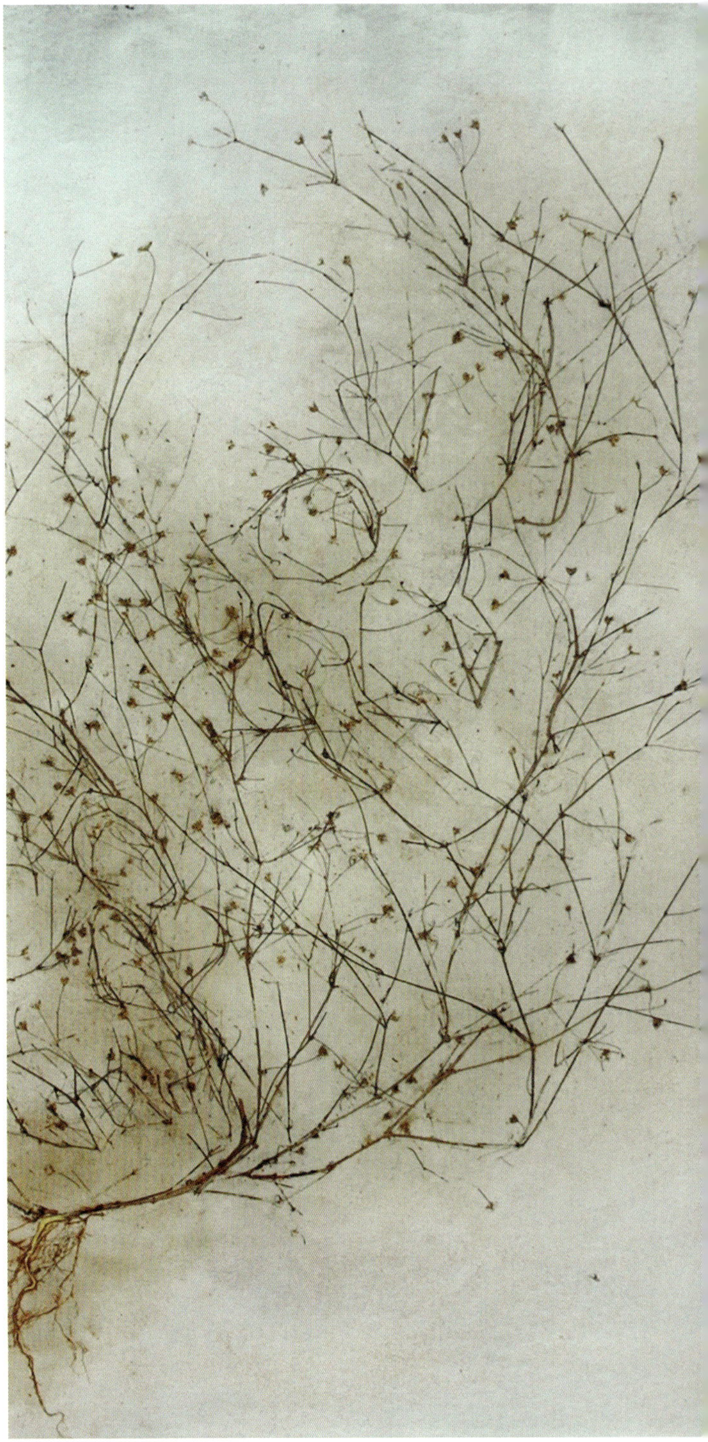

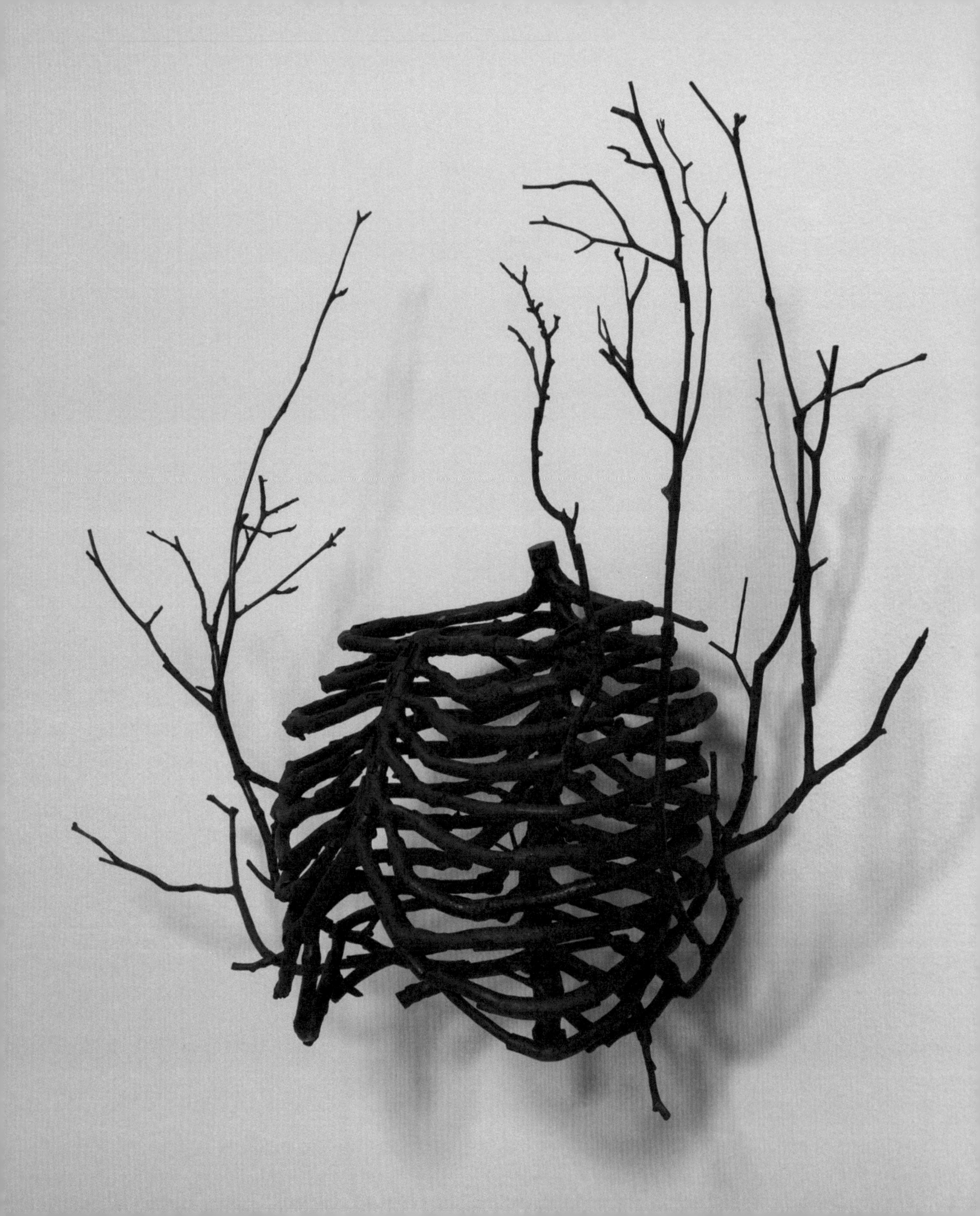

living people can be reconstructed, using the branching patterns of a tree, back to a common trunk: our most recent common female ancestor lived in Africa approximately 150,000 years ago (*see illustration: p 44*). So, human dispersal and migration can be mapped by following the direction of the changing patterns of mtDNA lineages. Similarly, we can map how paternity has contributed to shaping the gene pool of living people by examining the distribution of Y-chromosome DNA, which is a record of what fathers pass on to their sons.

PAGE 45: Gerhard Marx, *Father father/Mother mother*, plant matter, glue and watercolour on cotton paper, 57 x 75.5 cm (detail), 2008.

LEFT: Gerhard Marx, *Scion*, Bronze, 70 x 100 x 30 cm, (detail overleaf) 2011.

We inherit half the hereditary material that is packaged in our chromosomes from our mothers and the other half from our fathers. The 23 pairs of chromosomes comprise 22 pairs (numbered 1 to 22, one from each parent) called autosomes, and the remaining pair, which is made up of the sex chromosomes (XX in females and XY in males). However, the mtDNA and Y-chromosome DNA are matrilineally and patrilineally inherited respectively, and so are accurate markers for mapping the history of populations back to their origins.

Genetic mapping can thus provide data about the individual's connection to human evolutionary patterns, but it cannot provide insight into identity. It cannot tell us who we are. We nevertheless have an abiding fascination with the idea of knowing where and who we came from, and this idea is most graphically represented as a genealogical tree, or family tree.

Family trees, according to Marx,[10]

> sketch our genealogical dispersal, from the individual through the expanse of family relations into the infinity of the gene pool. This bifurcating branching structure follows the individual branch as it splits into the two separate branches that would represent the two parents and so it repeats, each individual owing its existence to two parents. The accumulation of this logic leads to the expansive complexity of the ancestral canopy, beyond which lack of knowledge makes it impossible to trace one's origins any further. But should one follow the directionality of this branch-logic, one would discover the problem inherent to the family tree: the genealogical tree grows into the past.
>
> The family tree grows from the present, the current individual into his/her ancestral past. It is perhaps logical that a structure concerned with the

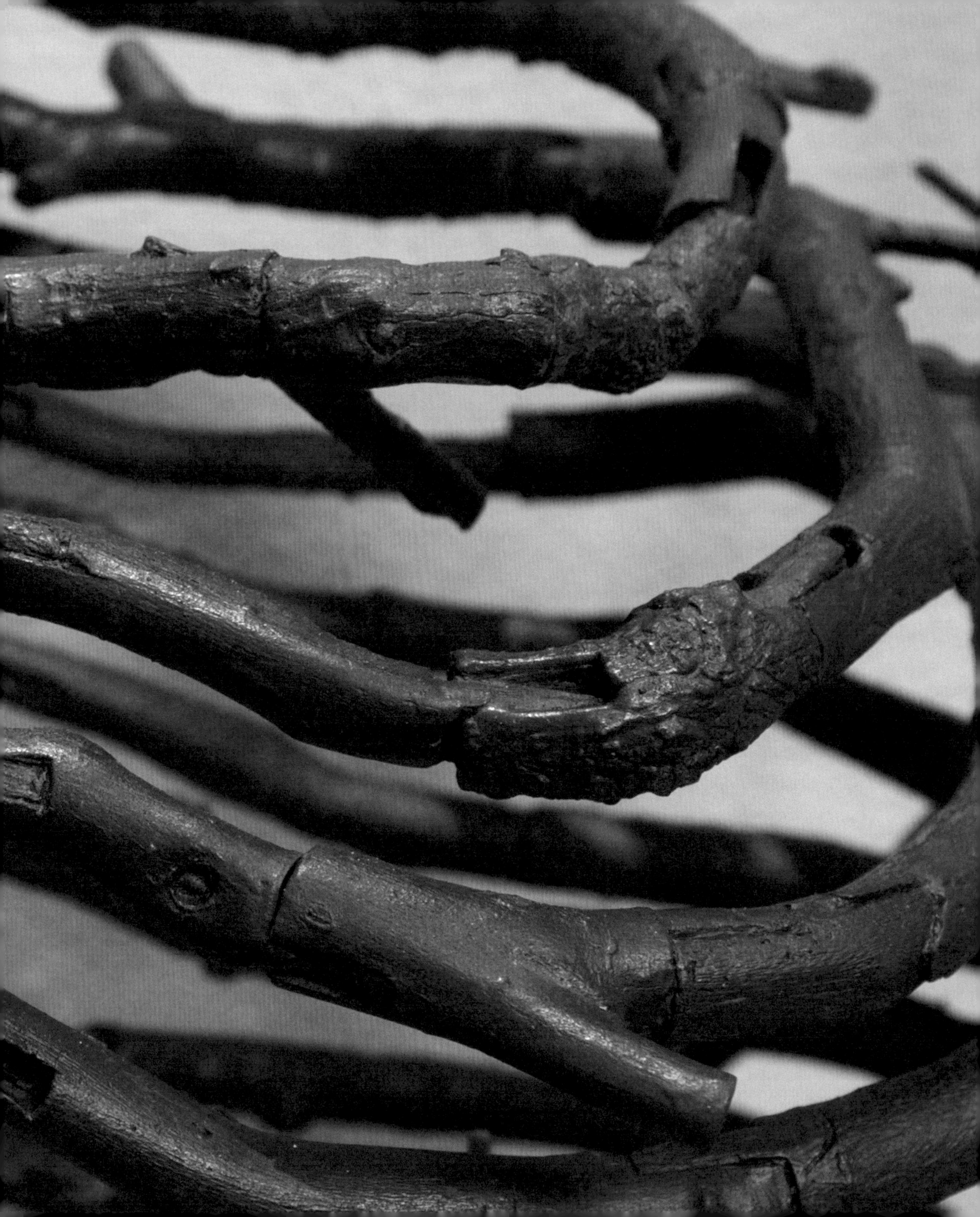

archive should grow like memory does; the branches spreading thin as its canopy expands. As long as the family tree operates as a mnemonic, archival device, the visual logic resembles that of an ordinary tree. But in truth the growth of the family extends into the continuous present through a directional logic that opposes that of the tree's growth. The growth-direction of the family tree funnels through the two branches of the parents, into the singular branch of the current individual, the current end of the line.

The direction of growth within the family tree opposes that of the real tree: it grows towards singularity as a type of unification rather than the bifurcation suggested by the image of the tree. The current individual is always the sum of two branches, but also always the end of the line – unless it is combined with another branch end. That new branch end is necessarily the logical end of a different branch, or tree structure. Try to imagine the tree as growing from its canopy to its base: you can imagine two branches becoming one (two parents giving birth to an individual), but unless growth stops there, another branch is needed for that branch to merge with to create another generation and so forth. The logic always ends with one, and another separate branch needs to be plucked out of the air, to merge with the current one.

In this sense, the growth-logic of the family tree is much closer to the logic of grafting than the natural growth of the mnemonic family tree. The family tree as one that grows into the present is one which grows through a continual logic of two becoming one, it is a tree that grows through the grafting of separate branches or trees onto each other to create a hybrid unity that will in turn need to be grafted onto another branch for its growth to continue.

The family tree only appears to grow as a tree when seen in retrospect, through the historical gaze, as a mnemonic structure. In reality, the family tree relies on a remarkably constructed, continued horticultural practice in order to continue its growth. The family tree (growing into the present), like any other tree, also grows into complexity, but that complexity does not lie in the density of its canopy. Rather, the complexity of the family tree lies in the endless hybridity of its grafted parts. Read in this direction, the singularity of the tree's stem is only the sum total of its vastly hybridised structure.

Many of us reflect on the past as a means of drawing strength for building the present and the future. We talk about our roots and of being rooted in our histories, an idea which has both productive and destructive dimensions. While we are all individuals who may carry the biological blueprint of many ancestors, our ideals are shaped in part by our environment and experiences, which is why issues of identity are so complex. When asked 'How do you identify yourself?', answers linked to race, nationality, culture and gender are possible, and there is no single answer to this question. Often, people expect that a genetic test can be used to tell them who they are. This is not the case. No genetic test can do that, but genetic ancestry testing (mtDNA in both males and females, and Y-chromosome DNA only in males) can be used to trace some parts of one's total genetic make-up. While this information forms only a small part of one's identity, it nevertheless has a tremendous impact on people yearning to understand their roots, and themselves.

The DNA approach to understanding human origins works backwards from a broad sampling of the genetic complexity of large, contemporary populations to a time when population was limited and homogeneous, establishing how an originating group split and evolved separately, becoming, over time, distinct populations. The importance of individual genealogy is subsumed by an interest in the patterns represented in the population.

For the individual interested in his/her forebears, the mapping works backwards, in geometric progression, from that single individual – the stem – to a myriad other individuals, from whom that person has stemmed. The primary focus here lies in the value of understanding a specific, individual origin, often used as an explanatory metaphor for identity. In such a family tree, the broader population patterns cannot be evident.

The aim of palaeoanthropology lies in creating a picture of human origins from fragmentary fossil evidence. Fossils are scrutinised for morphological changes to explain the development of biological structures in the present.

The impulse that compels people to seek answers about their origins from all these processes appears to be a global drive, a deeply human impulse. This impulse is variously represented – through papers with pie-charts and closely argued texts to computer printouts intelligible only to the initiated; from popularising cartoon narratives to abstract, conceptual works such as those done by the three *Life of bone* artists. Though so variously expressed, human consciousness seems to compel us to seek answers about our nature and our life paths.

The life of Sarah Bartmann ended in sorry circumstances in France, and her remains became the focus of a prurient, pseudo-scientific curiosity, driven by a socio-political need to demonstrate both superiority and otherness. The immediate fate of her mortal remains exposes the highly politicised nature of research, particularly that related to humankind's development. The occasion of her burial brought home to me the profound ways in which science is influenced, if not driven, by the social politics of the moment.

Notes

1 Sarah Bartmann, also known as the 'Hottentot Venus', was born in the Eastern Cape in the 1770s. She lived nearly three decades in South Africa, then spent some time in Europe, and died at the end of 1815. Following her death, Georges Cuvier, a revered scientist and comparative anatomist at the time, dissected her body, and her skeletal remains were measured and used as the type-specimen for Khoisan people. For more details on the life and times of Sarah Bartmann, see *Sara Baartman and the Hottentot Venus: A ghost story and a biography* by Clifton Crais and Pamela Scully, 2009.

2 The Reference Group (Department of Arts and Culture), a broadly representative ministerial advisory body that included representatives from the Khoisan community, academics, scientists, human rights practioners and advancers of gender/women's rights issues, were responsible for assisting the state with the interment of Bartmann's remains with dignity, compassion and sensitivity.

3 Diana Ferrus is a writer and performance poet. Her poem, *I have come to take you home – a tribute to Sarah Bartmann* was instrumental in the return of Bartmann's remains to South Africa. Ferrus is also a member of the Reference Group.

4 http://www.jrank.org/history/pages/6347/Neanderthals.html'>Neanderthals - Neanderthal Phylogenetic Status, Neanderthal Biology and Behavior, Neanderthal, Neandertaloid, Homo, Homo habilis, Homo erectus.

5 Gould observes that the holdings of the museum did not include female brains nor male genitalia. 1985. 'The Hottentot Venus' in *The Flamingo's smile*. New York: W.W Norton & Company. p. 292.

6 Bataille, G. 1993. *The Accursed Share: An Essay on General Economy, Volumes II & III*. Transl. Robert Hurley. New York: Zone. Quoted in Posel, D. and Gupta, P. (eds). 2009. 'The Life of the Corpse: Framing Reflections and Questions' in *African Studies*, December, 68(3), p. 302.

7 Posel, D. and Gupta, P. (eds). 2009. 'The Life of the Corpse: Framing Reflections and Questions' in *African Studies*, December, 68(3), p. 303.

8 Willan, B. 1984. *Sol Plaatje: a biography*. Johannesburg: Ravan. p. 4.

9 Mandela, N. 1994. *Long walk to freedom: the autobiography of Nelson Mandela*. Boston, New York, Toronto, London: Little, Brown and Company. pp. 3–7.

10 Some thoughts from Gerhard Marx on family trees: personal communication.

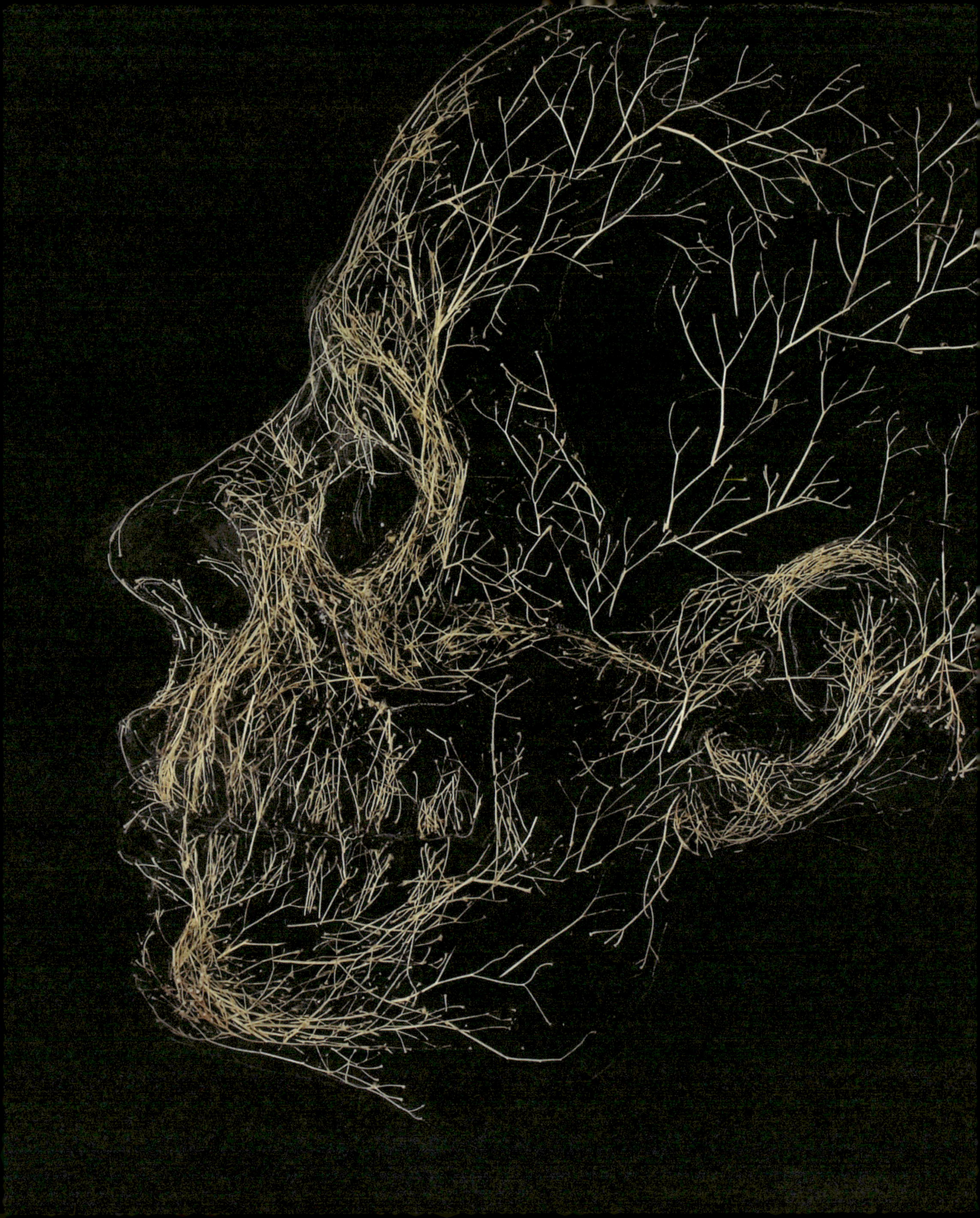

Chapter 3

Being-craft: Gerhard Marx

Elizabeth Burroughs

The riotous abundance bowled them both over on their return. The two-metre square of barren earth they'd managed to prize open before they left sported a shock of vivid green. After decades of being trapped, dormant beneath the concrete paving, the seeds had erupted, responding to the imperatives of earth, air, light and rain, and flourished. And so, instead of coming back to a desiccated enclosure, they were welcomed by this invasion. Unattended and unchallenged, the plants had made their comeback.

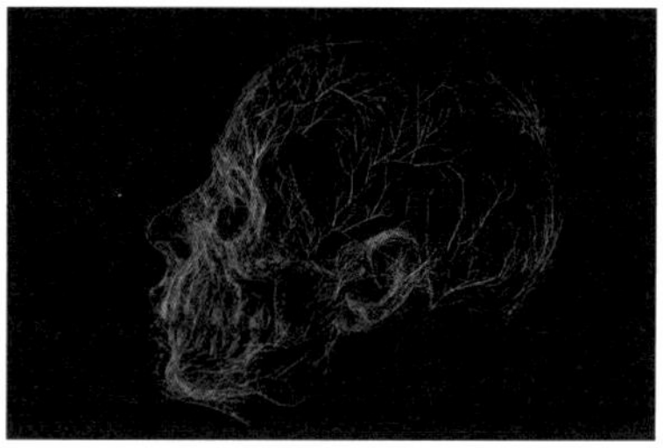

Gerhard Marx, *Weeds II*, plant material, watercolour and glue on cotton paper, 92 x 142 cm (detail left), 2007. Johannesburg Art Gallery.

This invasion of their space took Gerhard by surprise – the plants had shot up within the boundaries he had thought secure, and yet, here they were. They made him feel fallible. He recognised there was something powerful to be learned from this subversive energy, and, as he pulled up the weeds – there were other plans in place after all – he began to appreciate their delicate toughness. The roots, from which he shook the reddish dirt, filled space like miniature branches. He fell in love with the repeated architecture of stem, twig and twiglet, the same patterns again and again on a different scale. Interest piqued, he knew there was something here that was precious enough to work with, though it was not yet clear how. Driven by an impulse to preserve these forceful presences, he dried them between sheets of newspaper.

Dried weeds burst out of the bath in the Melville flat that serves as Gerhard's studio. The various plant sorts provide different kinds of line. With a practised eye, he knows which roots to snip, and which stems, for the work in hand. Leaves, he says, don't survive the adhesion-and-abrasion process particularly well. He takes the selection back to the worktable. The pot of cold-glue with its paintbrush, the roll of wax paper, and the bone folder lie on the drawing he is working on. A rib is there too. And beyond, on the counter, a couple of sturdy femurs lie crossed.

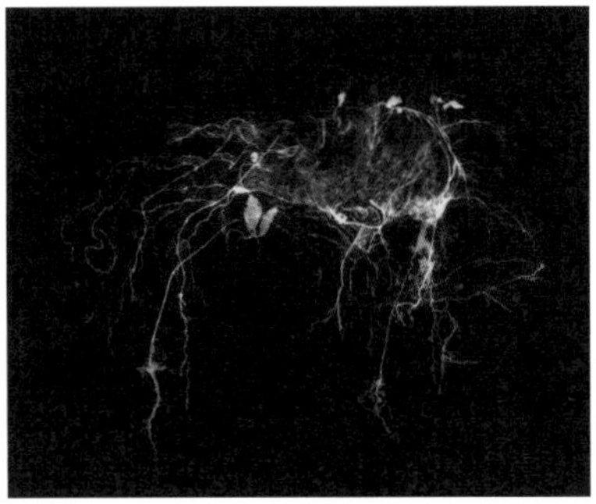

Gerhard Marx, *Grandmother with weeds*, photographic contact print, 48.5 x 58.5 cm (detail right), 2007.

With a quick check at the rib, he amends the pencil line on the drawing, and then scans the dried sticks and rootlets for the best approximation to the line. The match is checked and then the glue is applied on an area about four centimetres square. He tears off a piece of wax paper big enough to cover it. Then, with deft fingers, he lays the plant matter along the line. Here the stem is gently tensioned to follow the line more exactly. Here the natural tendrils are allowed to extend organically beyond the pencil mark. The left hand hovers with the wax paper at the ready for the moment when the fit is right, then applies it with a practised firmness. The bone folder looks just like a well-used sliver of soap and is critical to the process because of its smooth hardness. Gerhard rubs the little area he has worked on with vigour, annealing plant material, glue and paper, and then whips off the wax paper before it also affixes itself. The folder, a relic from another age when paper was folded and cut by hand, is the essential tool here, though he had no idea how he might use it when he bought it at Talas in New York, the least expensive thing in the whole shop. If he can't find the whalebone folder in the productive disorder, he may as well not work. The next stalk is chosen, laid down on the glue to make the line, covered and burnished. And then the next – one careful iteration follows the next.

Sorting out a new technique – the *how* of managing the materials to work with and for him – form the first steps of the creative process. Finding expression through the particular technique then facilitates ways of being in the world that were not there before. Weeds, perhaps regarded at most as a recurrent irritation in the making of a garden previously, have been seen afresh as expressing the very thrust of life – in Dylan Thomas's phrase, 'the force that through the green fuse drives the flower'. They become a potent source of new perception, not just of themselves, but of ideas that connect, that serve to re-represent the world.

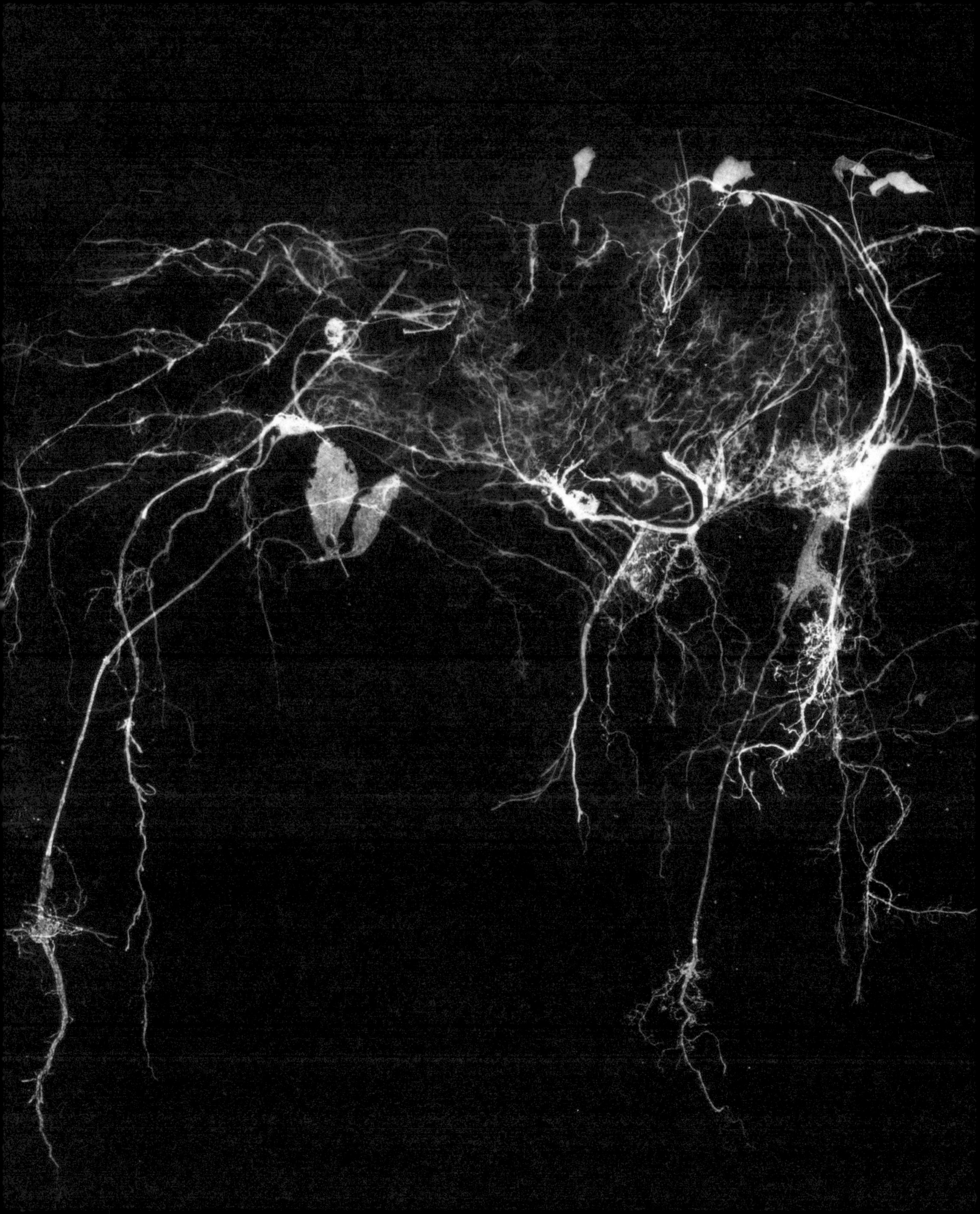

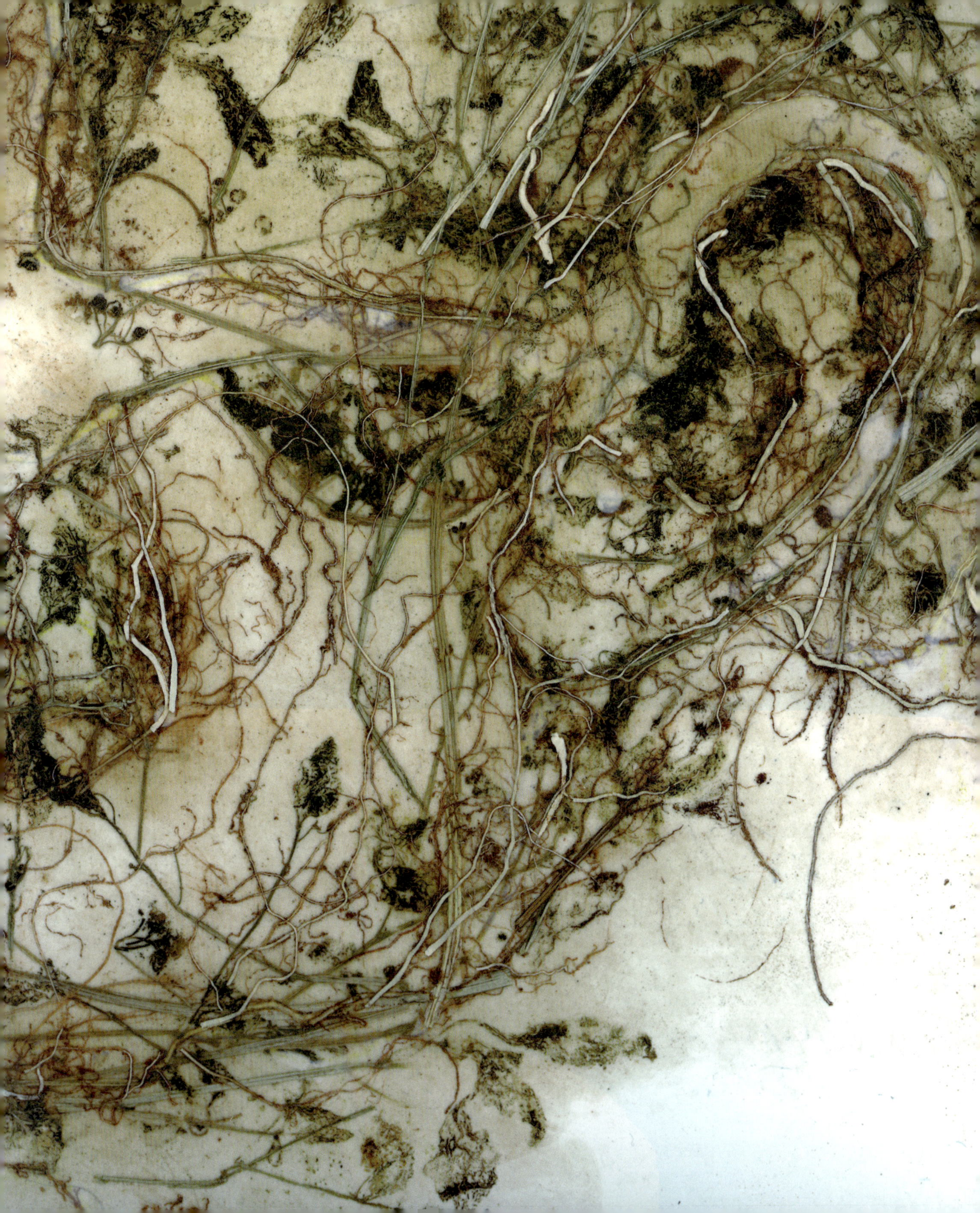

The glued sections are almost dry. The process is helped along with the blast of a hair-dryer, and then, with an electric tool that looks like an iron, Gerhard sands the image down to a silky flatness. Where pencil once intimated form, now the fractals of red rootlets do the defining. A small section of a nameless plant creates a mark in shades of grey and taupe. The ribs and skulls in the drawing – for it still belongs to that tradition of making – are bone, but alive with growth. Pared down to within a few microns, these plant segments, gathered in interstitial urban spaces, challenge us to consider their lives as well as the bigger picture which usually nullifies their significance. We see the skulls, ribs and femurs, but we also see the structure of the plant stems that define those forms, moving perpetually between levels of perception.

The use of dried plant matter as the technology for poetically embodying thought-provoking works inevitably results in rich networks of association. Gerhard knows – and continues to be amazed by the fact – that the first actual preservation of plant materials as a record by Luca Ghini was a relatively late phenomenon. His *Hortus siccus,* a dried garden preserved in a book, was compiled in 1544, fifty years after the first printed books of woodcut illustrations of plants had created vigorous interest in matters botanical. As Gerhard says, it was as if the plants themselves only became real to viewers once they had been represented. In a sense, his works form part of that *hortus siccus* tradition, except that the technique of the preservation of the plant on paper serves different goals: the death of the plants gives life to fecund images. From the merest traceries of roots and leaves, for example, he evokes a portrait, which is an image of himself and of the archetypal figure of the green man, both friend and foe, whose life transcends death cyclically.

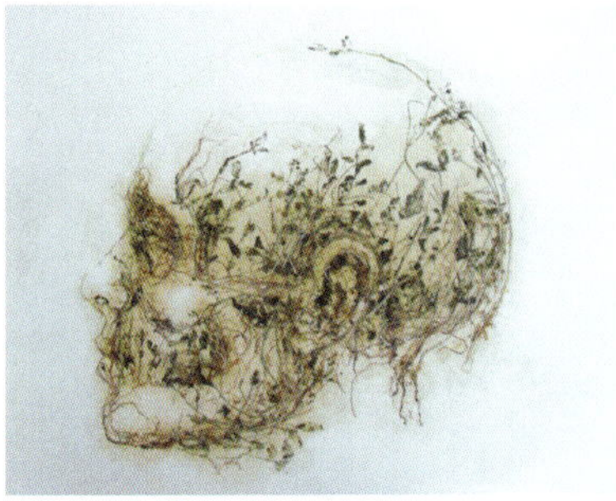

Gerhard Marx, *Weeds IV*, plant material, watercolour and glue on cotton paper, 47 x 65 cm (detail left), 2008.

The places where Gerhard harvests the weeds that form the raw materials for his work are neglected sidewalks and vacant plots. These are where – in Manley Hopkins' words –'weeds in wheels grow long and lovely and lush'. Like the outlawed plants that flourish in these spaces, so too do desperate humans whose lives are just as liminal as those of the plants. Collecting there means going out of one's safety zone and into places where violence may lurk. While Gerhard clearly does not regard his work as overtly political, the subject matter of bones emerging amongst the weeds talks – though with a different voice – as much about the violence that characterised our past as it does about threat in the present. The concerns are similar to those expressed in Himla Soodyall's paper on bones and genes and in Kopano Ratele's writing when he connects Joni Brenner's paintings to the traumas manifested in the TRC hearings. And, while Joni's work seems to partake of the fantastic energy that Giacometti saw was needed to sustain life, Gerhard's is about the fabulous, horrific beauty of bodily collapse, the dissolution of form and function when that energy runs out. He intimates that our consciousness of the here and now, our normal consciousness, is Gothic, perforated as it is by a violent past and saturated with crime.

Born in the catalytic year of 1976, Gerhard matriculated in 1994, the year of the first democratic elections in South Africa. With his early life bracketed by such critical events, it is inevitable that his experience of that history should determine how he would relate to the world around him. He comments that as a young Afrikaner man, the only relationship to himself possible was ironical, not fertile ground for the creative, but one which has resulted in his work pointing to the genotype rather than the phenotype, a preference for the indexical which points away from the self. This looking at the deep structures rather than at the surface ones has allowed for a much more acute phenomenological approach to being in the world, a world which involutes itself into the mapping of what it means to be human.

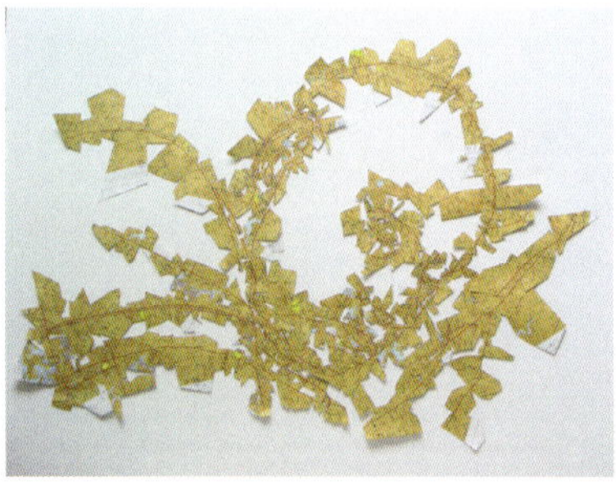

Gerhard Marx, *#6 (Grandfather)*, cut and reconstituted map fragments, 123 x 89 cm (detail right), 2003. SANLAM Collection

And so, Gerhard is also a gatherer and hoarder of maps, and to that end, he haunts second-hand bookshops where he buys old atlases. The colouration used in older maps is more subtle and satisfactory, but maps from different eras all have a different appeal. The use of snippets of maps to create portraits preceded the use of plant matter, and required the development of a technique that allowed him to handle the tiny fragments without getting glue on them. In these works, he chooses a small stretch of roadway that corresponds to the contours he has laid down as a draft before he begins. Excised from the map with a scalpel and ruler, the piece is glued in place so that – in time – the original drawing is completely covered, concealed by the red and blue lines, while the territory that comes with them begins to represent flesh or bone. Once the entire image has been created by this meticulous process, it is carefully separated, stroke by scalpel stroke, from the paper on which the image has been laid down. The defining lines of the

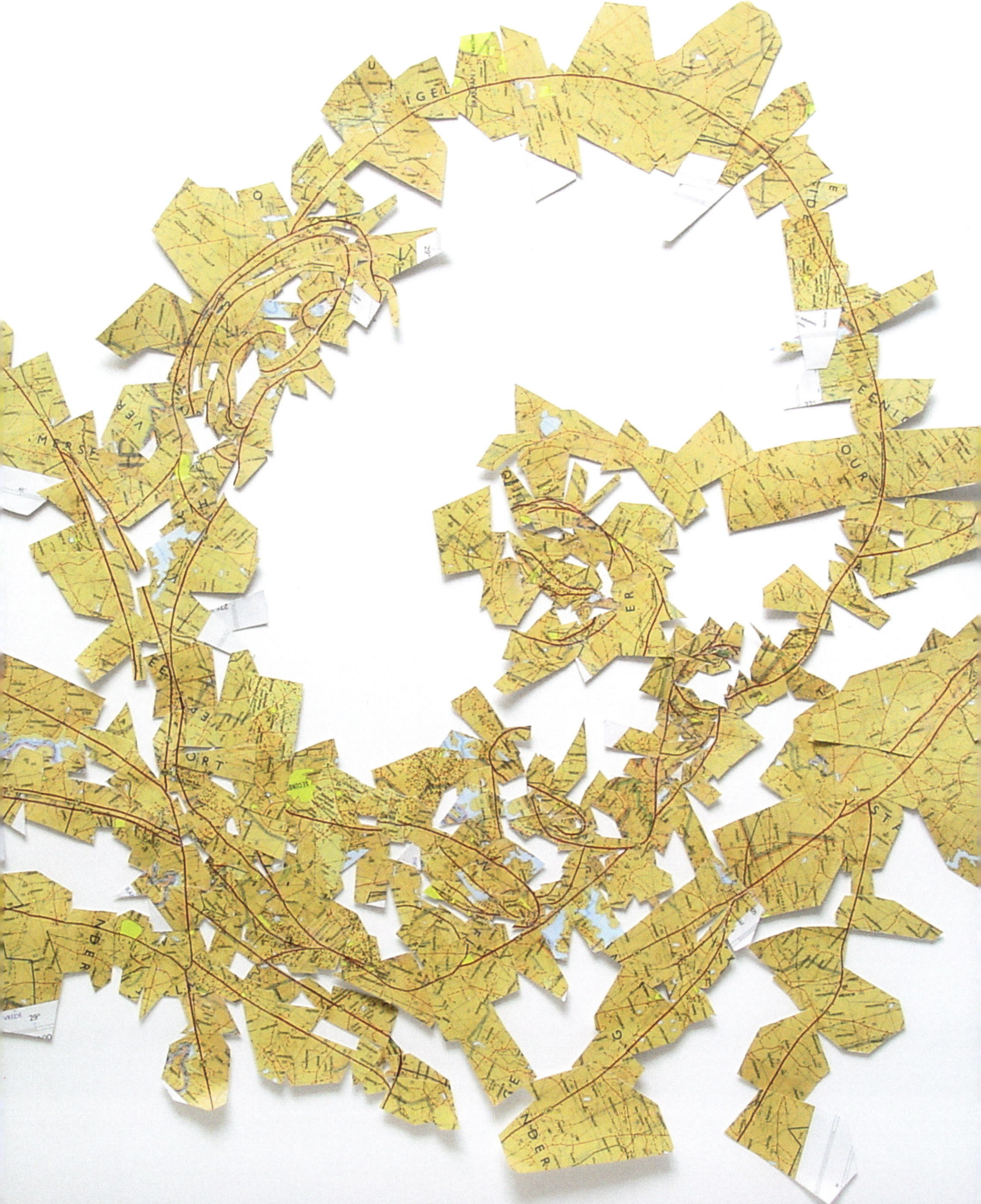

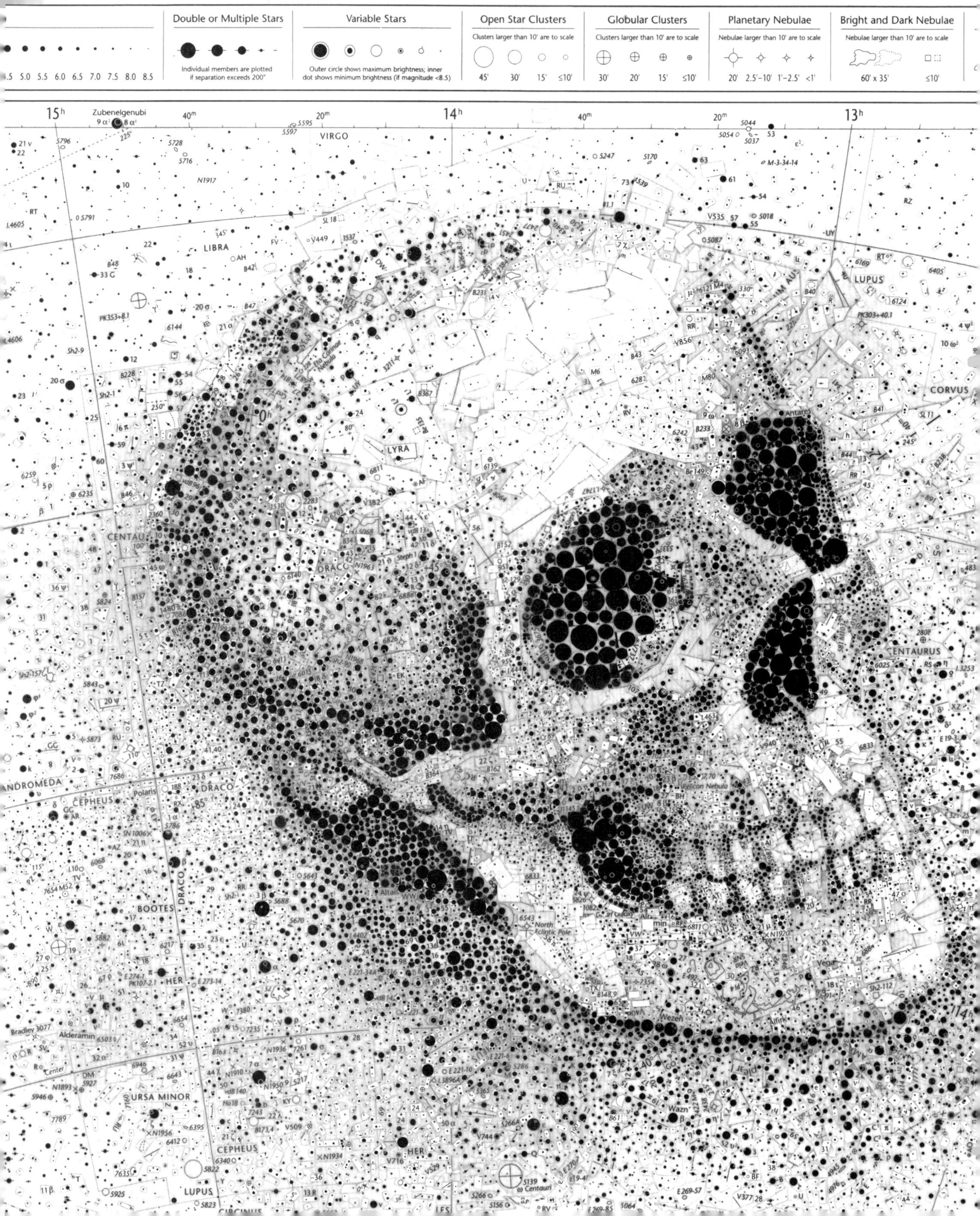

Double or Multiple Stars
Individual members are plotted if separation exceeds 200"
Variable Stars
Outer circle shows maximum brightness; inner dot shows minimum brightness (if magnitude <8.5)
Open Star Clusters
Clusters larger than 10' are to scale
45' 30' 15' ≤10'
Globular Clusters
Clusters larger than 10' are to scale
30' 20' 15' ≤10'
Planetary Nebulae
Nebulae larger than 10' are to scale
20' 2.5'–10' 1'–2.5' <1'
Bright and Dark Nebulae
Nebulae larger than 10' are to scale
60' x 35' ≤10'
5.0 5.5 6.0 6.5 7.0 7.5 8.0 8.5
15h 40m 20m 14h 40m 20m 13h
Zubenelgenubi
VIRGO
LIBRA
LUPUS
CORVUS
LYRA
DRACO
CENTAURUS
ANDROMEDA
CEPHEUS
Polaris
BOOTES
HER
URSA MINOR
Alderamin
Antares
Pelican Nebula
North Ecliptic Pole
Vega
Wezen
Wazn
ω Centauri

portraits read also as arteries and veins, suggesting an external and internal view simultaneously. This process, which gives a whole new meaning to cutting and pasting, takes time: a skull made up of thousands of black dots, representing stars of different sizes, is set against a star map. This small work took a year to construct. The result is breathtaking, but the point is that the revelation, the uncovering has happened in the doing. It is in contemplating the stored labour that we begin to understand the wealth of the connections Gerhard is making. In such doing, he understands what it is to be, but the works are also, in the Heideggerian sense, a sending that invites us to see for ourselves what these visual texts disclose. The map points to the territory but is not it. And Gerhard's maps of the body, of the mind, radically dislocate the world as we know it, not cynically but lovingly.

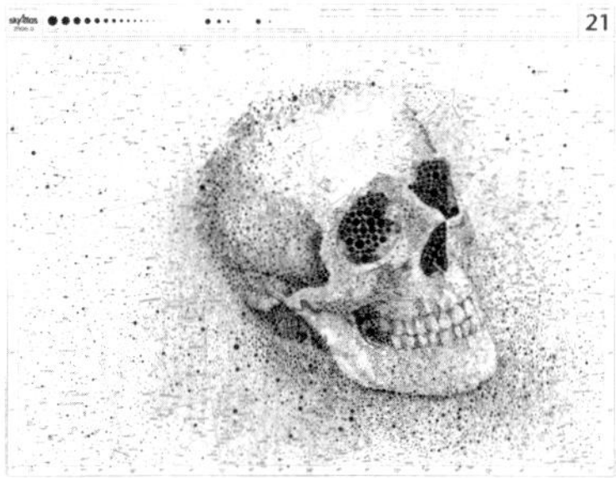

Gerhard Marx, *Dark Sky* (right hand panel of triptych), cut and reconstituted map fragments, 34.2 x 46.6 cm (detail left), 2007. The Marvellous Collection.

Gerhard sometimes talks about fighting the works he is doing: a new series, based on that most mobile and mercurial of forms – cumulus clouds – is being put together using a most fixed and seemingly inflexible medium – black 30-centimetre rulers. The sculptural work has a sleek core of black wood as its base, and stacked against this, in serried ranks, the rulers mount up to suggest the shifting tumult. He shows me earlier versions where he heated the rulers virtually to melting point to get them to flow in curves, almost poisoning himself with the fumes in the process. The solution has a grace and simplicity that is compelling and hard won.

The use of the maps and rulers for purposes other than the ones they were intended for suggests that the conceptual underpinning embodied by these objects – these technologies – have a role to play in the reading of the works, and so it shouldn't come as a surprise that the loaded South African place name, Weenen, can be discovered close to the eye in one work. The rulers, which are placed against other rulers, touch each other, not some other object which is measurable by this proximity, somehow resulting in a collapse of purpose. The fine lines and numerals seem to suggest shimmering cloud linings. Rulers, all measurement, he says, were based on the proportions of the body: the inch, the foot, the ell, and so the rulers, which have to touch the thing they measure, approximate skin, the largest organ of sensation. The natural, the human and the technical brush up against one another in a way that is both restrained and passionate.

Past and present perpetually brush up against one another in Gerhard's

Gerhard Marx, *Dark Sky* (right hand panel of triptych), cut and reconstituted map fragments, 34.2 x 46.6 cm (detail), 2007. The Marvellous Collection.

work too. His thinking about how the past is concealed in the present emerges so clearly in his writing about the conventional interpretation of family trees, where, he argues, the directional logic is misleading, causing the current generation to be seen as the outermost tips of the highest branches. He argues instead that, in some senses at least, the current individual is, in the present, the ultimate stem of endless sets of graftings that grow backwards in time: a multiplicity of ancestors find their singularity in the latest scion of the line.

We speak about Gerhard's experience of fatherhood, a dissolution of the body, he calls it. 'It's a collapse of the singularity of the body, for it is as though part of you is walking outside of yourself. It's as if one's skin has dissolved and there has been an expansion beyond the boundaries of the body. The self is no longer singular.' He has shifted from being trunk to branch, still part of the tree, but he has moved upward towards the multiplicity of branches.

It is little surprise then that, when asked to write for the *Beeld* about an artist who has influenced his own work, Gerhard chose Guiseppe Penone, the Italian sculptor. The sculptures which Gerhard analysed are felled trees, which Penone has pared away until he has revealed the much younger self of the tree concealed within. Unlike other living beings, trees preserve their younger incarnations within their present form, meaning that one can whittle away later accretions and still find the younger form of the tree intact, which is exactly what Penone has done. I think Gerhard's fascination is as much with Penone's ideas as with the forensic precision that the sculptor must use to bring forth the *alethia*, the truthful representation of the earlier tree. Penone's work has the same respectful relationship to the material he works with that I recognise in Gerhard's work. The making process discloses the way both artists relate to the things of the world: their approach could not be more radically different from, say, the way of knowing and being revealed in Georg Baselitz's *Ding mit Arm,* brutally chainsawed from a linden tree. Artists are both knowers and do-ers, who challenge others by letting the structures of existence be seen, things that sometimes resist being seen, as Gerhard has observed:

> Human remains, particularly bone, are an object-type that I think of as self-effacing. These are objects (like maps, photos, fossils) that operate in a totally

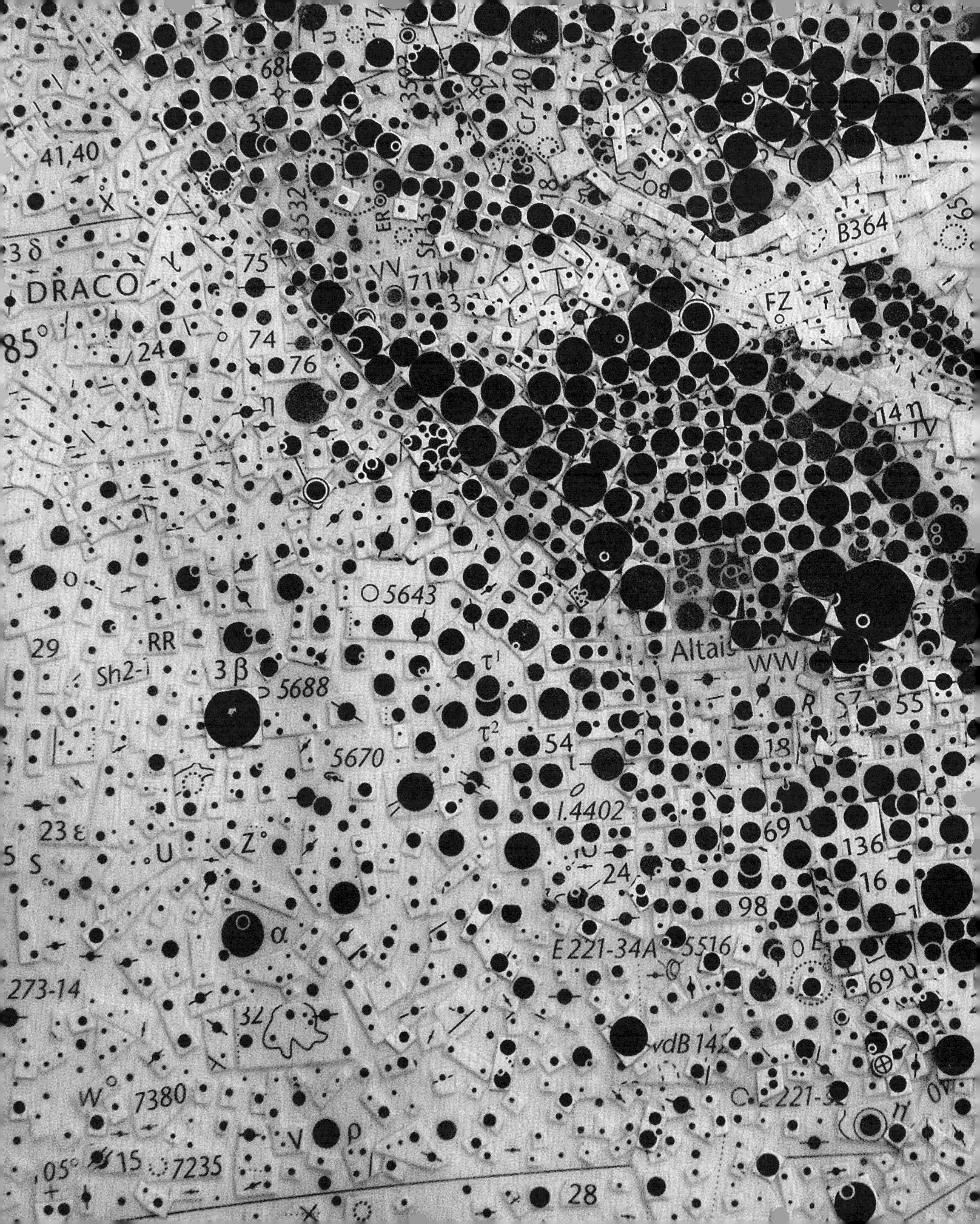
41,40
DRACO
85°
75
74
76
24
71
VV
Cr 240
B364
FZ
14 η
5643
Altais
WW
29
RR
Sh2-
3 β
5688
τ¹
τ²
55
54
5670
18
I.4402
69 υ
136
23 ε
U
Z
24
16
98
α
E221-34A
5516
273-14
vdB 142
W
7380
V
ρ
05°
15
7235
28

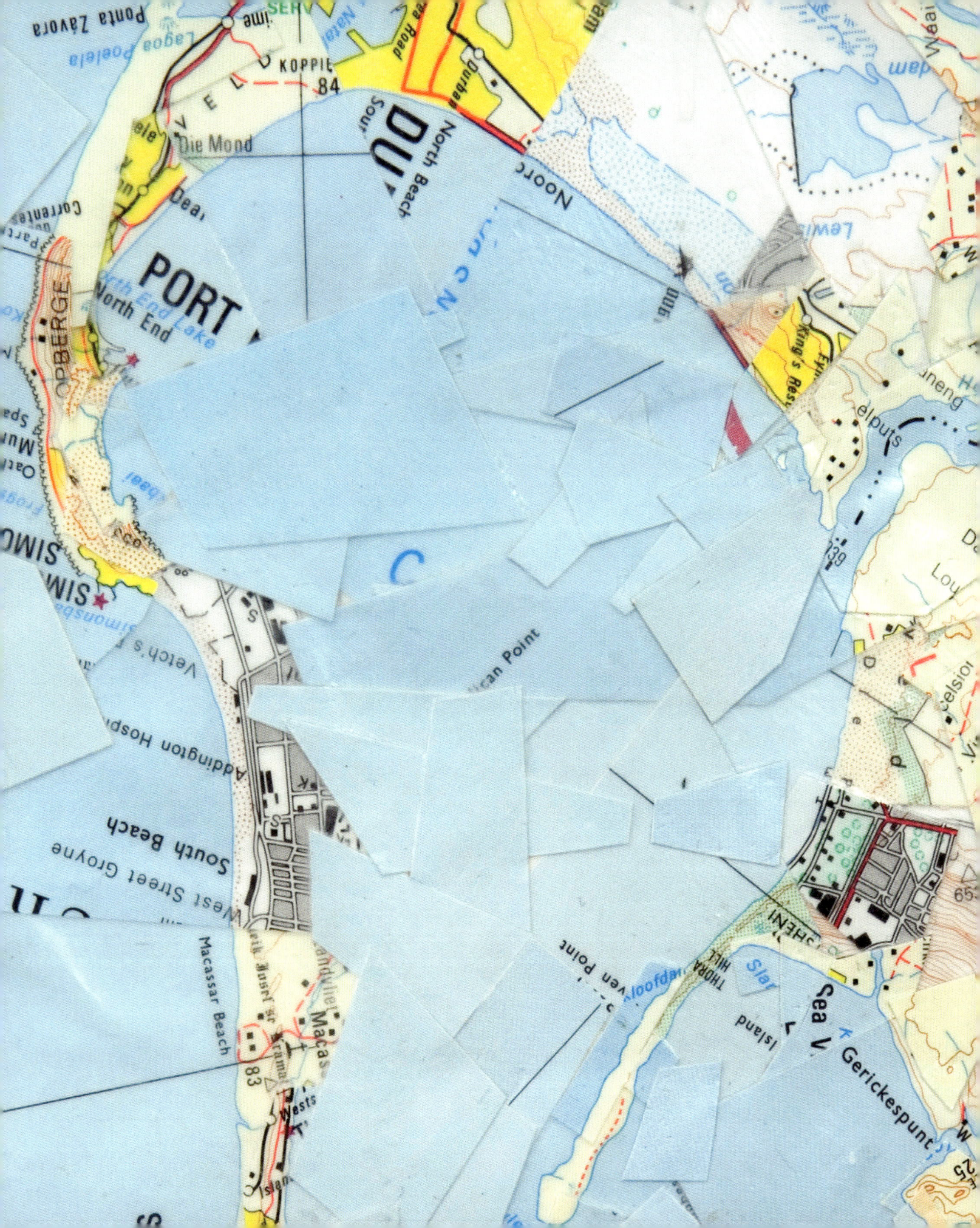

Ponta Zavora
Lagoa Poelela
KOPPIE
84
Die Mond
North Beach
PORT
North End
North End Lake
Lewis
ican Point
Vetch's
Addington Hosp
South Beach
West Street Groyne
Macassar Beach
83
THORA HILL
Island
Sea V
Gerickespunt

indexical manner. This category of object always, unfailingly points away from itself, towards an exteriority, towards an event that has taken place elsewhere, a place outside, a life that was. The insistence with which these objects point away from themselves obsessively negates their own presence, to a degree of near invisibility. This invisibility is arrived at through the object's ability and determination to camouflage itself in allusion.

Though Gerhard here refers to objects which are the subjects of his works – or the medium which he uses to construct them, this description could apply to the works themselves: the real referent is alluded to, and the real location of the work resides in the mind of the viewer.

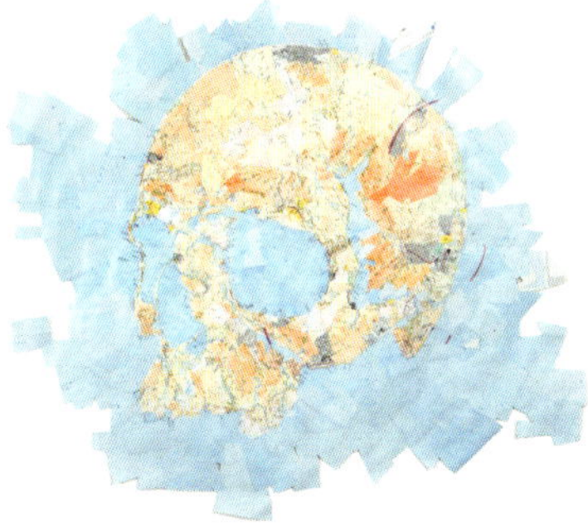

Gerhard Marx, *Aggregate skull II*, cut and reconstituted map fragments, 123.5 x 123.5 cm (detail left), 2010.

As I leave Gerhard's flat, elated by the hours of talking and looking, I pass Ira Bekker's studio on the corner. She is putting together a *Cave canem* mosaic I recognise from my standard six Latin textbook. She has spent all afternoon neatly placing hundreds of small tesserae down to form the background. It's clear that there are days of similar work ahead. And yet, from piles of black and off-white ceramic bits, her labour has brought into being a dog on a chain. She has worked steadily at her craft, revealing beauty that was not there before. I think how lucky the people are who will get to live with that hound with his red collar.

As it turns out, I wrote the first part of this piece about Gerhard by hand, something I've not done in years: I was in Cape Town without my laptop, but so wanted to start. Writing is always a slow process for me, regardless of the technology, but writing by hand was more like choosing the right piece of weed and getting it down on paper. I'd forgotten the crossings-out of false starts, the words inserted afterwards, the arrows moving a section of text from one place to another. It reminded me that writing on the computer is just one way in which I could write, not the only way. Writing by hand felt a bit more like laying down the words one by one, like tesserae or bits of map, allowing these words on Gerhard's work to come in the hope that I might reveal my truth about the nature of his work, and what I have learned from him.

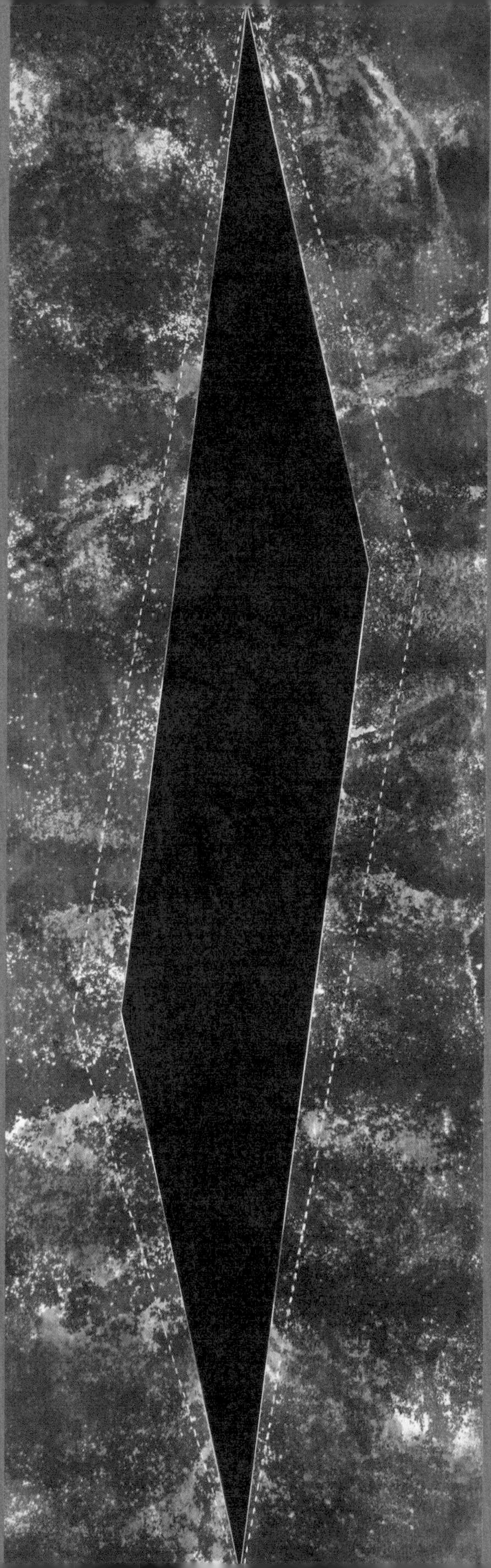

Chapter 4

Part of the story

Kopano Ratele

> My work over decades has explored the interface between the seen and the unseen, the known and the unknown, between the graspable and the elusive, between certainty and uncertainty. As an artist, I am constantly thrown back on the uncertainty of perception, of things not being what they appear to be, always grappling with the challenge of finding a mode of representation that is at once defined and ambiguous. These seams between the clear and the unclear, or between knowledge and intuition are focal in my work. They are also strongly central to the investigative probing nature, and the construction of symbolic language systems, devised by scientists. It is clear that artists and scientists constantly work and teeter on the outer limits of knowledge and comprehension, and that both embrace similar febrile strategies to engage their insights. This understanding of scientists is contrary to generally held perceptions that science is emphatic knowledge that does not tolerate ambiguity; this dead certainty was long given its authority by a political and theological order that authorised such knowledge as singular, sanctified and sure. But it is also a defensive knowledge that reacts against and resists rival knowledge.[1] Whereas science has traditionally been seen as objective, and art as merely subjective, my work on this project in particular deflates the authority of these polarised views. In some ways, the works emerge equally from a sense of comprehension and of incomprehension.
>
> Karel Nel, *Disrupted knowledge*[2]

Karel Nel, *Leaping darkness*, sprayed pigment on bonded fibre fabric, 250 x 80 cm, 2008

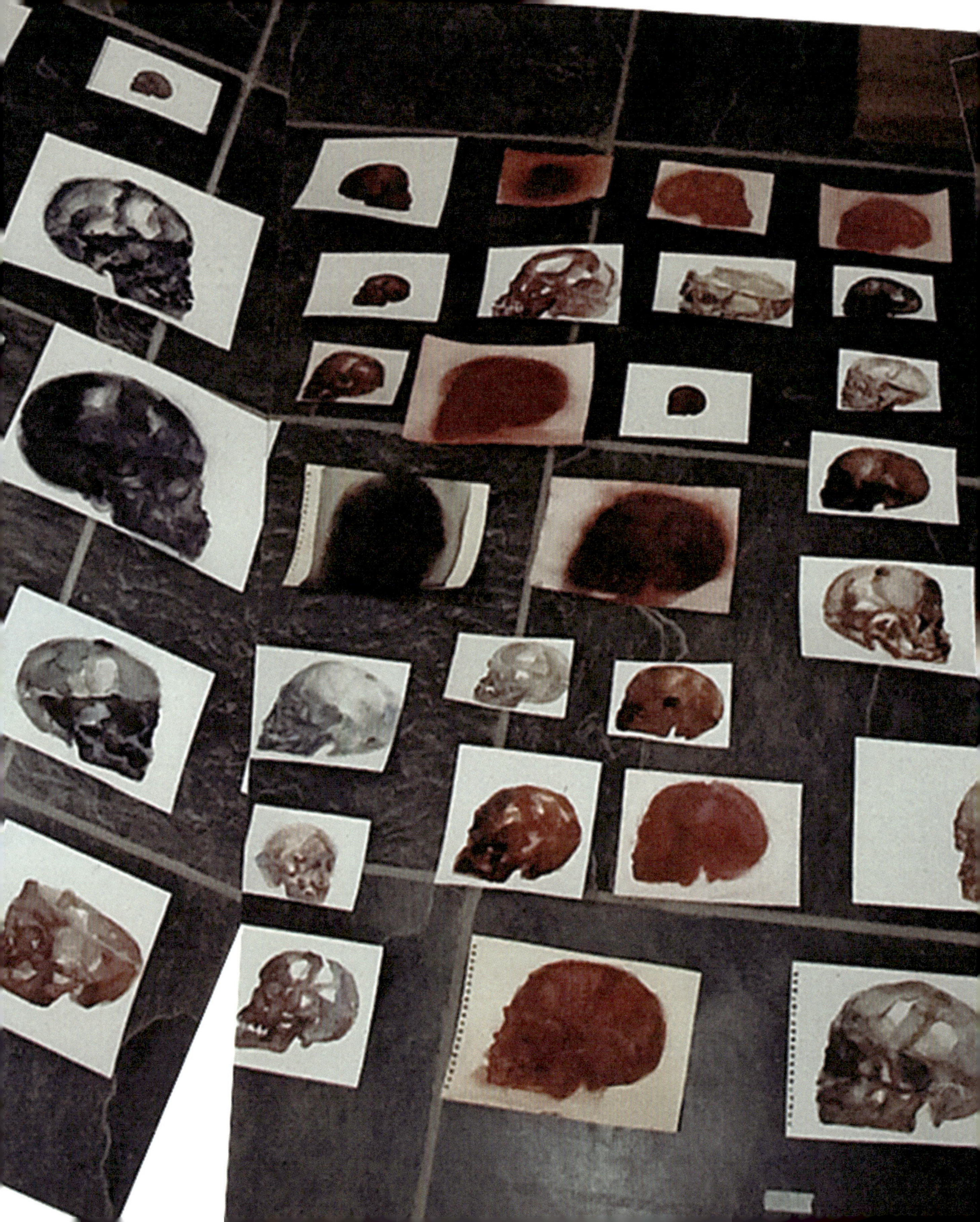

Even though it is part of the fabric of daily life, the inevitable incompleteness of knowledge is unsettling to many of us. While we desire to know all of the truth about a moment in a day that we feel is important, or a life and its end or origins, sooner or later we come to realise that we can never be totally confident or satisfied with what we find. But Joni Brenner is the artist of uncertainty. Like Karel Nel, Brenner is attuned to things being other than what they seem. That may be one reason that Nel's work is one of the two other artists' work that Brenner wanted alongside her own in the *Life of bone* project.

In my estimate, an artist of uncertainty, like Brenner, does not imply one who is uncertain about the world around her, for the politics of a country such as hers, and the history of violence that has characterised it, can induce feelings of uncertainty in most: it certainly does not mean doubt about what she paints or sculpts. The contrary is true: she paints this very uncertainty. It appears to impel her to reveal a fractal reality in her work, rather than to retreat from the unknown, ambiguous and elusive, that Nel too seeks to represent. As she says about the redness of some of the watercolour skulls and some of the oils too, redness represents both the red of violence and the red of the life force. In her obsessive skull-making, in both paint and clay, her work is a constant study on what it is to be human. Art is a process of discovery of her subject, of getting to the story, more than merely aiming to represent. As she noted in one of our exchanges:

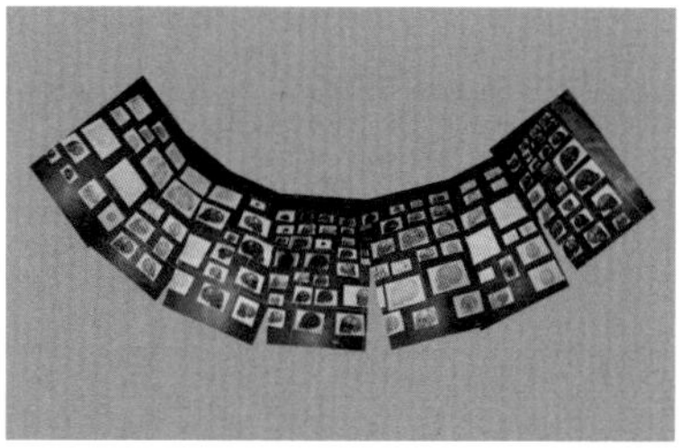

Joni Brenner, Maquette for installation of *Wall of skulls*, composite photographs, 26 x 64 cm (detail left), 2011.

> My skull-work, and the unending repetition, is partly to do with a meditation on life/death and what is and is not present in bones/skulls. Like any representation, the skull is a physical presence, and confirms an absence. Skulls or remains can tell only part of a story. There is so much unknown and unknowable. Perhaps to fit this into a broader picture, the search for knowledge, for truth of some kind, is at the heart of scientific and artistic pursuits. The focus on remains, on the skull, is, in part, a focus on the past, on origins, on seeing the past in terms of the present or the present in terms of the past. Looking much further back, these same issues are attached to my work with the Taung child's skull.

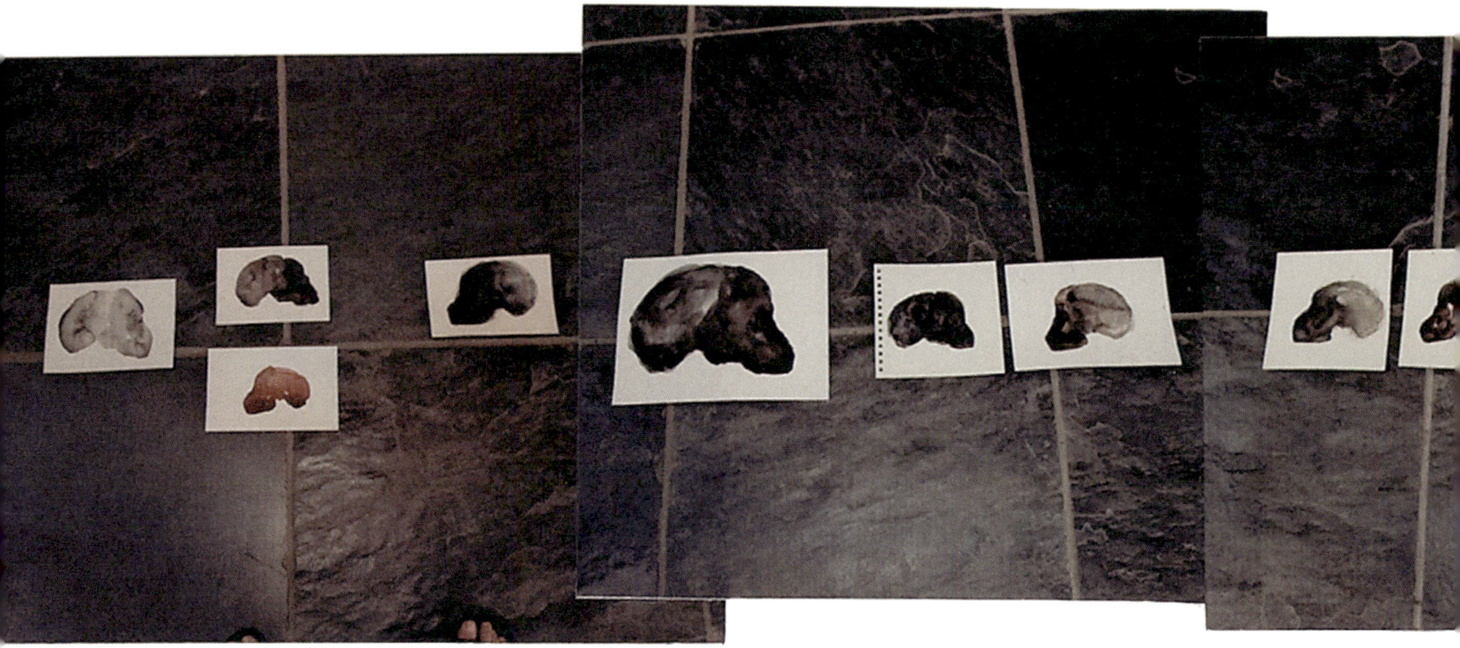

More generally, the uncertainty that underpins Brenner's work is expressive of the fact that a project, a painting, a journal article – she is also an art historian – or even a building is never really done. In science, as in art, there is no true end, one merely pauses between one moment and the next, and between one question and another. While for some people there is satisfaction with having finished a piece of work, for others the work is never done until it leaves the studio, gets sold, is installed elsewhere, or published. Even then, someone like Brenner always recognises the work may have turned out differently, that it shouldn't have gone the way it did, that it will always be unfinished. This is what she was to say to me about her own work, but I think also more generally about art and science: that she finds that there is an elusive element about knowing, portraying, imagining others, a need to work with the material over and over.

Joni Brenner, Maquette for installation of *Taung series*, composite photographs, 12 x 54 cm, 2011.

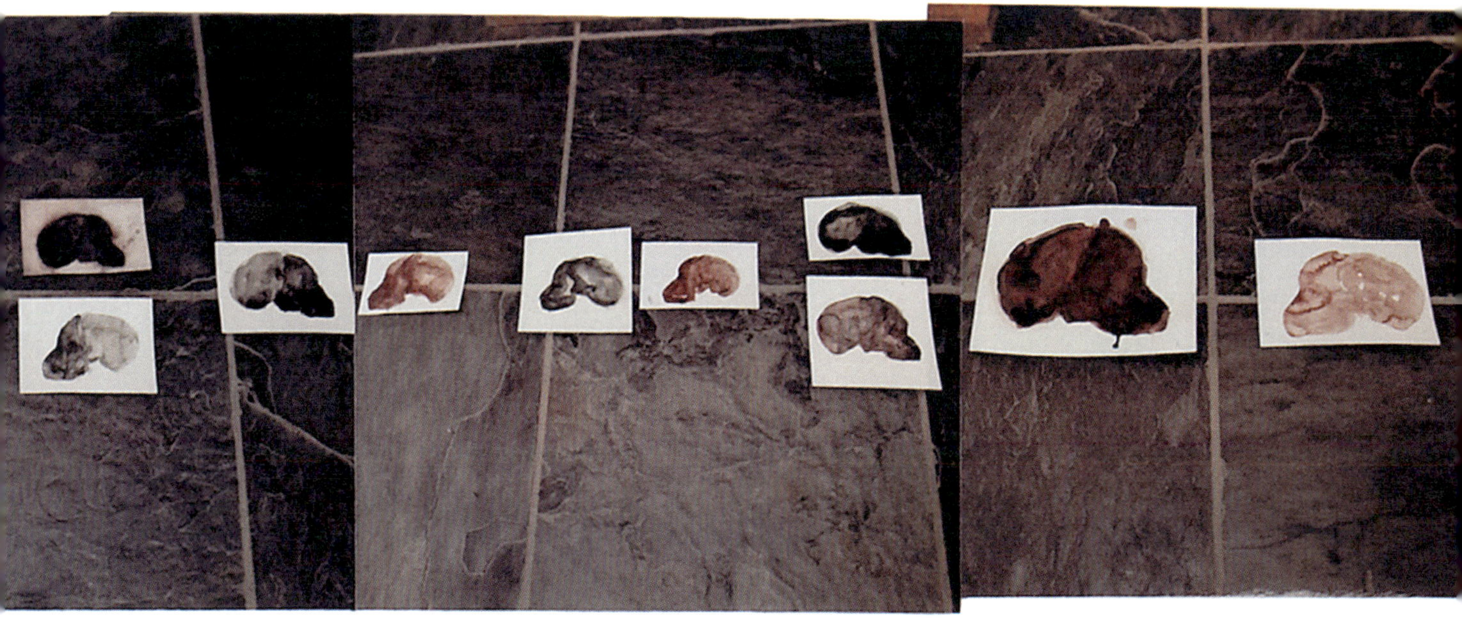

Although we intuit that we can never fully grasp all about an event in the past, we still long to know everything about it. Probably, that is the central ontological dilemma of science. At the same time, it is also the inspiration for further enquiry. We are above all driven to find out about our own lives and the world we live in because we do recognise that nothing can ever fully and elegantly answer the questions we have; that nothing can extinguish all the uncertainty about why whatever happened took place – one's own birth being a quintessential example here. The resolution of this discomfiting knowledge is to admit that, as Brenner's skulls appear to indicate, bones do have life. Something remains after the last breath, after decomposition even. It's an odd thing, but her skull work expresses that there is untrappable energy in the past, that there is, as it were, life in the Taung skull and other bones.

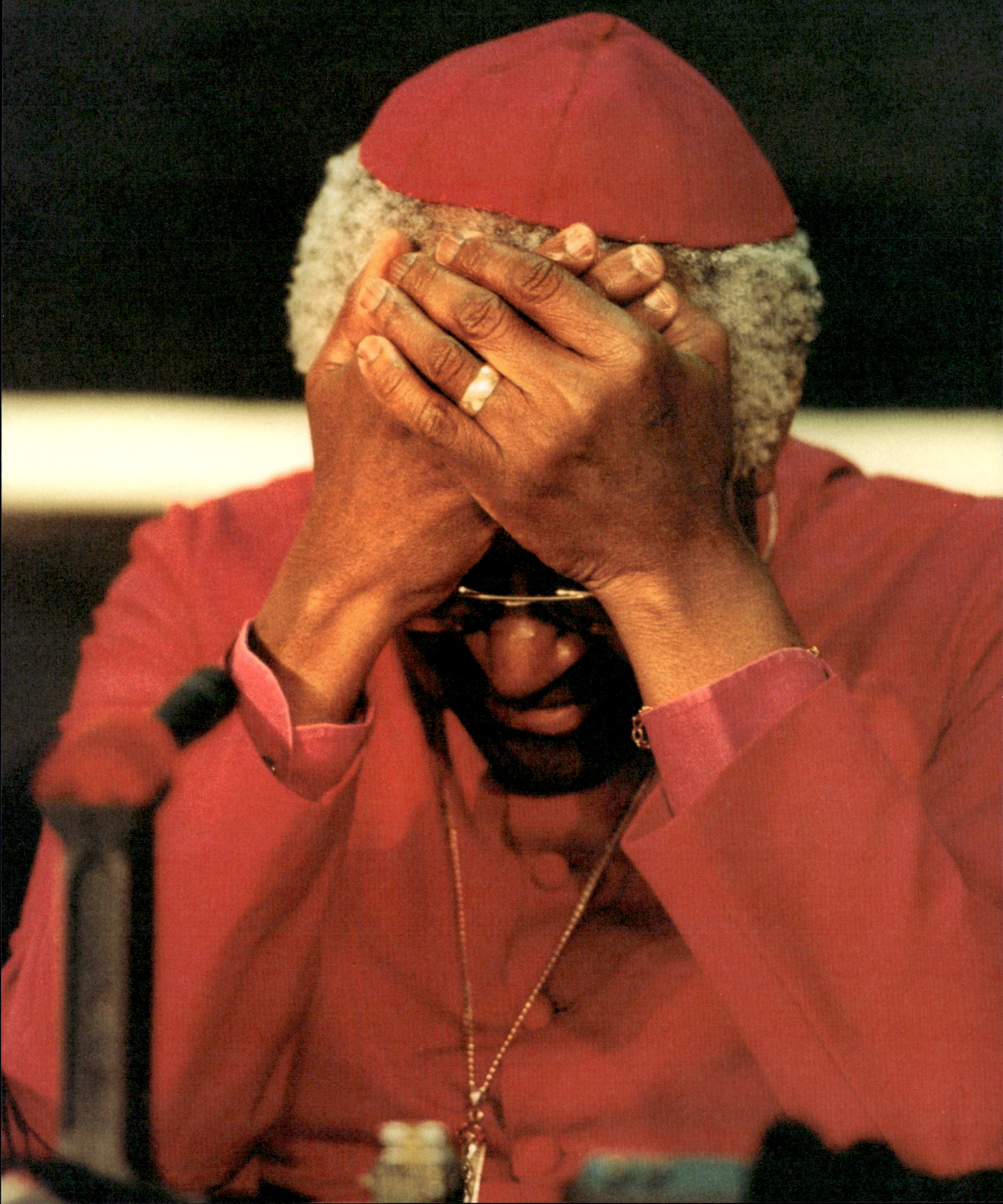

It may not be surprising to her, but it is to me, that this uncontainable energy is also to be glimpsed at work in that defining moment of recent South African history: the Truth and Reconciliation Commission (TRC). It may be that the TRC was about this very need to find reassurance in the face of what one senses can never be fully settled. The past refuses to be buried, returning to haunt the present, changing it in multiple observable and unseen ways.

It is true that the stated objectives of the Commission were said to be the promotion of national unity and reconciliation in a spirit of understanding which transcends the conflicts and divisions of the past by – a) establishing as complete a picture as possible of the causes, nature and extent of the gross violations of human rights which were committed during the period from I March 1960 to the cut-off date, including the antecedents, circumstances, factors and contexts of such violations, as well as the perspectives of the victims and the motives and perspectives of the persons responsible for the commission of the violations, by conducting investigations and holding hearings; b) facilitating the granting of amnesty to persons who make full disclosure of all the relevant facts relating to acts associated with a political objective and comply with the requirements of this Act; c) establishing and making known the fate or whereabouts of victims and by restoring the human and civil dignity of such victims by granting them an opportunity to relate their own accounts of the violations of which they are the victims, and by recommending reparation measures in respect of them.[3]

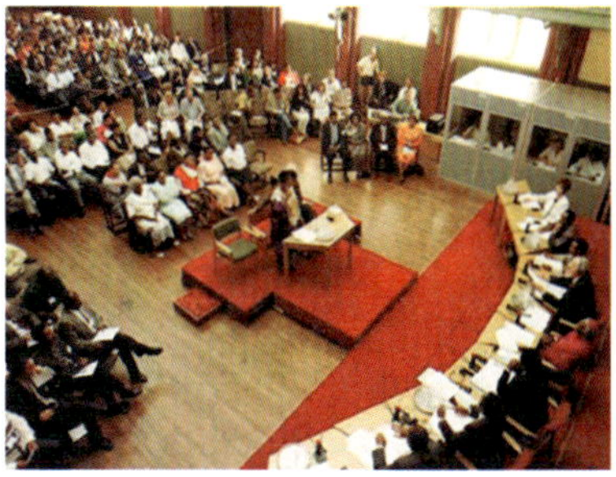

General view of the TRC Commissioners and the hearing underway. The person giving testimony is Nobuhle Hilary Mohapi, the very first person to give public testimony before the TRC in East London on 15 April 1996. She was detained and tortured in 1977 following the arrest of Steve Biko for whom she worked as a secretary. Photograph by Rob White, courtesy iAfrika Photos, 1996.

However, an unacknowledged wish of the TRC was the desire to bring, as René Descartes had it, true and certain knowledge to a history of trauma. On the basis of such truth, it was hoped we would be able to reconcile ourselves with the past as much as with one another. Then again, the TRC must have appreciated that telling about a deeply distressing event must be imprecise, which is the reason there was a need for corroborating evidence for those who gave testimony.

Archbishop Desmond Tutu breaks down in tears while listening to the testimony to the TRC of a man who was tortured by the apartheid security police. Photograph by Raymond Preston, courtesy *Sunday Times*, 1996.

Evidence for the possibility that there was, behind the TRC's creation, a desire to bring certainty regarding a painful past can be found in several places. One of

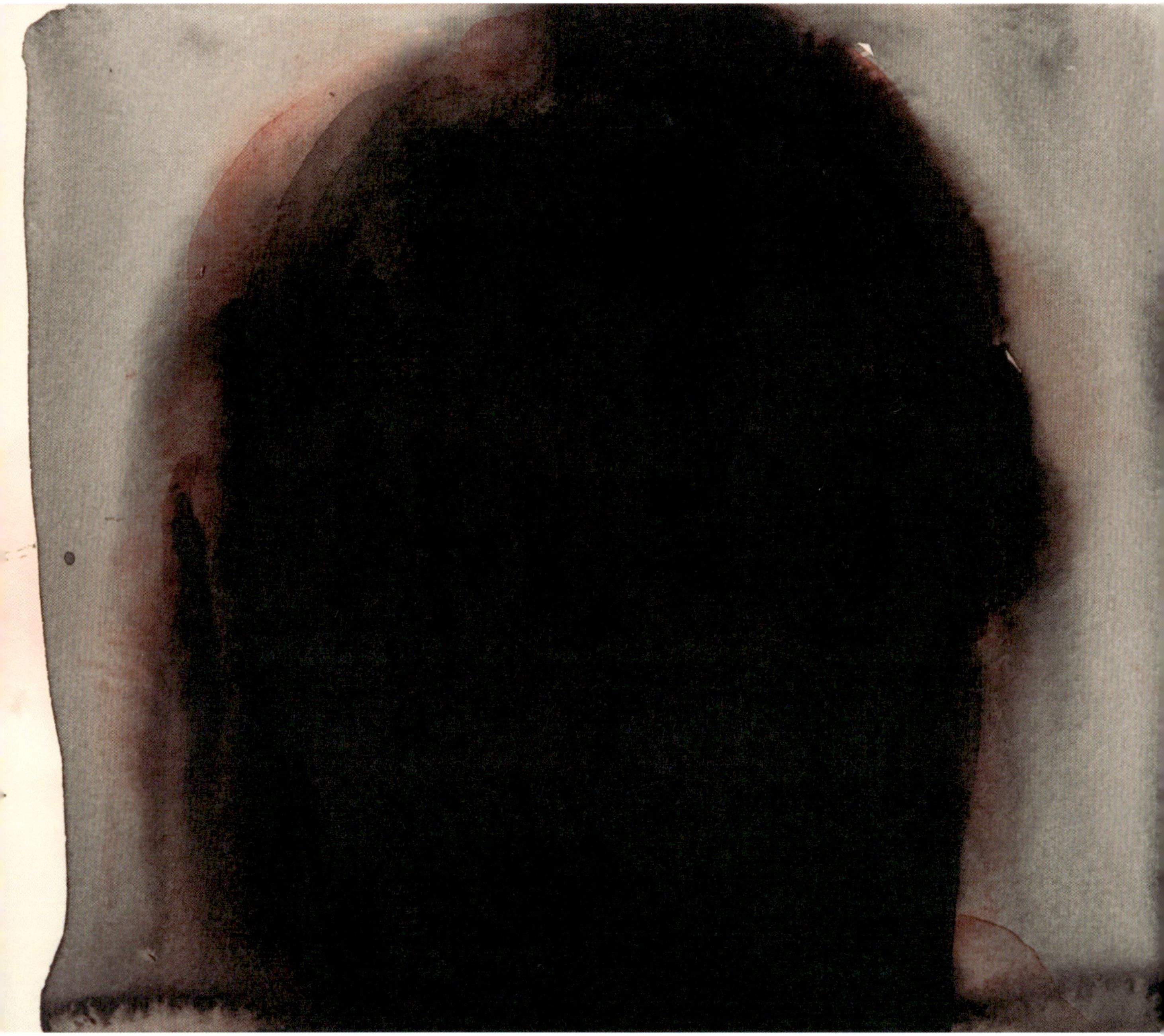

these is the TRC Final Report's chapter on reconciliation. In that chapter, the TRC adduces select moments from the life of the Commission as indicative of 'significant steps in the reconciliation process'.[4] The work undertaken by Hugo van der Merwe on Duduza in the wake of a hearing in that township is referred to:

> Victims are not ready to engage in a reconciliation process unless they know more about what happened. They often say they are willing to forgive, but they need to know who to forgive and what they are forgiving them for. A willingness to reconcile is dependent on people's ability to cope with and process their knowledge of what had happened. While the past remains hidden, a reconciliation process proceeds on very shaky foundations. The [Commission] has contributed to some of this revealing, but many individual victims are still in the dark about the details of their specific cases.[5]

Part of the need to 'know more about what happened' was the longing to find out where the bones of one's family or comrades were buried. Archbishop Desmond Tutu, who chaired the TRC, recalls how 'at one of our hearings a mother cried out plaintively, "Please can't you bring back even just a bone of my child so that I can bury him." This is something we have been able to do for some families and thereby enabled them to experience closure'.[6]

Looking for and finding the bones of those we once knew, for some people at least, helps to reduce the level of uncertainty, which was invariably experienced as traumatic. This ability of bones to debunk constructed counter-realities and to allow one to take cognisance of the past is further attested to in Volume 3, Chapter 6, of the TRC Report, which speaks of the death of Stanza Bopape, a well-known name from the archives of anti-apartheid activism. Before his death, Bopape held the position of general secretary of the Mamelodi Civic Association. He died while in the custody of the South African security police in 1988, three days after he had been detained:

Joni Brenner, from *Wall of skulls,* watercolour on paper, 17.5 x 25 cm, 2010.

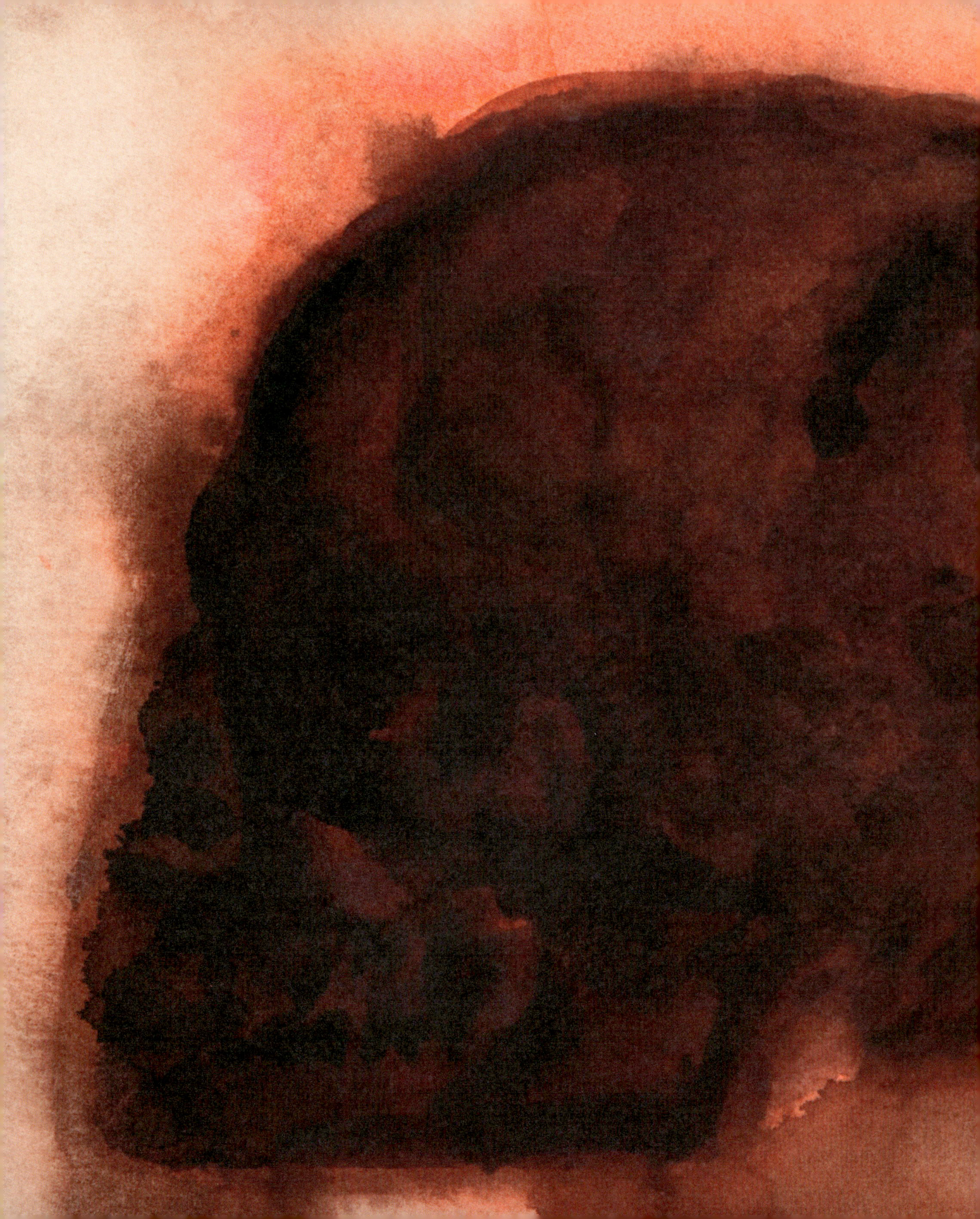

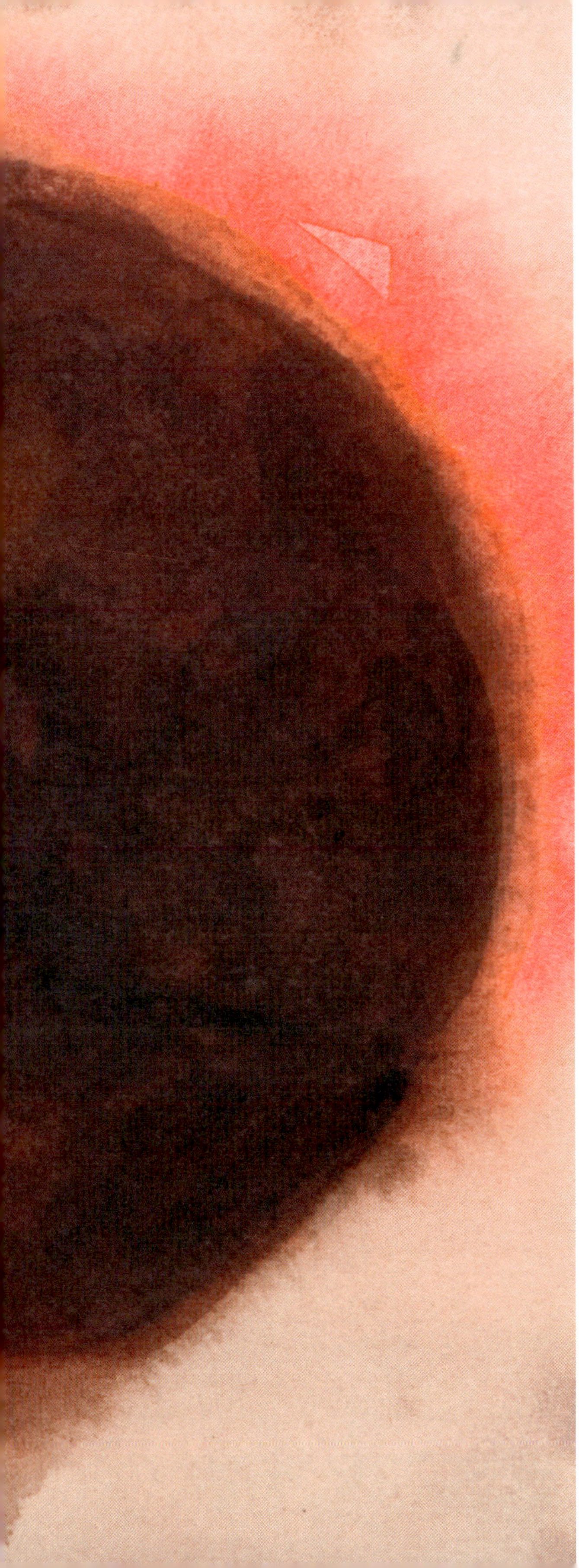

> A high-level cover-up, including a fake escape and secret disposal of Mr Bopape's body was approved by the commissioner of police, General Johan van der Merwe, in order to avoid the negative political ramifications of his death in police custody. Until the recent amnesty applications of a number of policemen involved in Bopape's death, a public fiction had been maintained that Bopape 'escaped' from police custody while being transported from Johannesburg to the Vaal. According to then-Minister of Law and Order, Mr Adriaan Vlok, Bopape escaped when three policemen with whom he was travelling got out of the car to change a punctured tyre. Bopape allegedly found the keys to unlock his handcuffs and fled. Police reported that they shot at him but failed to apprehend him, and claimed that he must have left the country to join the ANC.[7]

Stories such as this about the workings of the apartheid state are now common knowledge. It is not the coldness that can be read here, or the murder, or its cover-up that is of interest for us now. Rather, it is Bopape's mother's recorded words at the TRC hearings in the last sentence below that move us:

> Mr Bopape's mother, Ms Mokgaetji Francina Bopape, breaking down several times, made an impassioned plea at the Commission's Pietersburg hearings for information about her son's whereabouts. After a fruitless search by her husband for Bopape in the ANC exile community, Ms Bopape became convinced that her son had died in police custody. However,

PAGE 76: Joni Brenner, from *Wall of skulls*, watercolour on paper, 18 x 26 cm, 2010.

> she was never able to confirm this. She told the Commission that she wanted 'the police who were with him [to] come here and tell us where the bones are' (620–621).[8]

Ms Bopape seemed to be saying that if only she knew where the bones were she would know something of significance for her own life and that of her family. Knowing where the bones were would be psychologically significant, perhaps because the hoped-for knowledge held the possibility of changing the meaning she and her clan gave to their lives. Brenner's comment on the *Life of bone* project, that we look backwards in order to re-see and re-make the past and shape the present, may just as well have been a response to the search by Ms Bopape for her son's bones. Ultimately, like Ms Bopape and others, we wish to exhume graves or search in morgues and hospitals for the bodies or bones of our children, spouses, lovers or comrades so as to help us stitch together our knowledge of the past and make sense of the present.

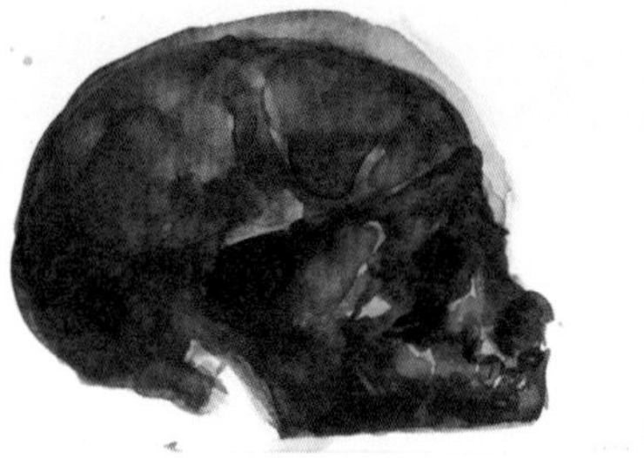

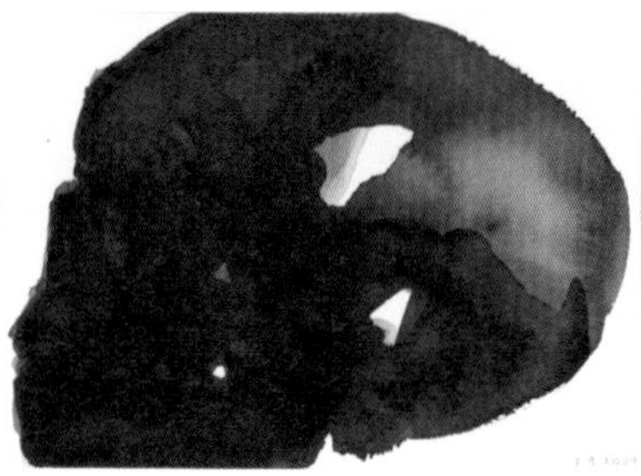

ABOVE: Joni Brenner, from *Wall of skulls*, watercolour on paper, 23 x 30.5 cm, 2010.

BELOW: Joni Brenner, from *Wall of skulls*, watercolour on paper, 14.5 x 21cm, 2009.

RIGHT: Joni Brenner, from *Wall of skulls*, watercolour on paper, 14.5 x 21 cm, 2009.

I am not sure whether there is a deliberate intention to do so, but Brenner's skull work also appears to seek to come to terms with the trauma of the past. When this aspect of her work is pointed out, her response is that one can't live in a place like South Africa without violence and abuse and pain, murder, torture and death, being a core part of one's mental furniture. The TRC as an event is, of course, just part of a continuum that is still unresolved: we can't live here without thinking about Boipatong, Sharpeville and the many secreted away events of our country – those that emerged in the TRC hearings, those that continue to emerge and to take place.

The manner in which she expresses her South Africanness is most instructive to me about her living and working, her being and being an artist, and is where I see the connection between her skulls and the trauma that is never too far under the skin of South African identification:

> My thoughts about my skulls and trauma/vulnerability settle . . . on the process of their making: daily, ongoing, unresolved or incomplete, incomplete-able.

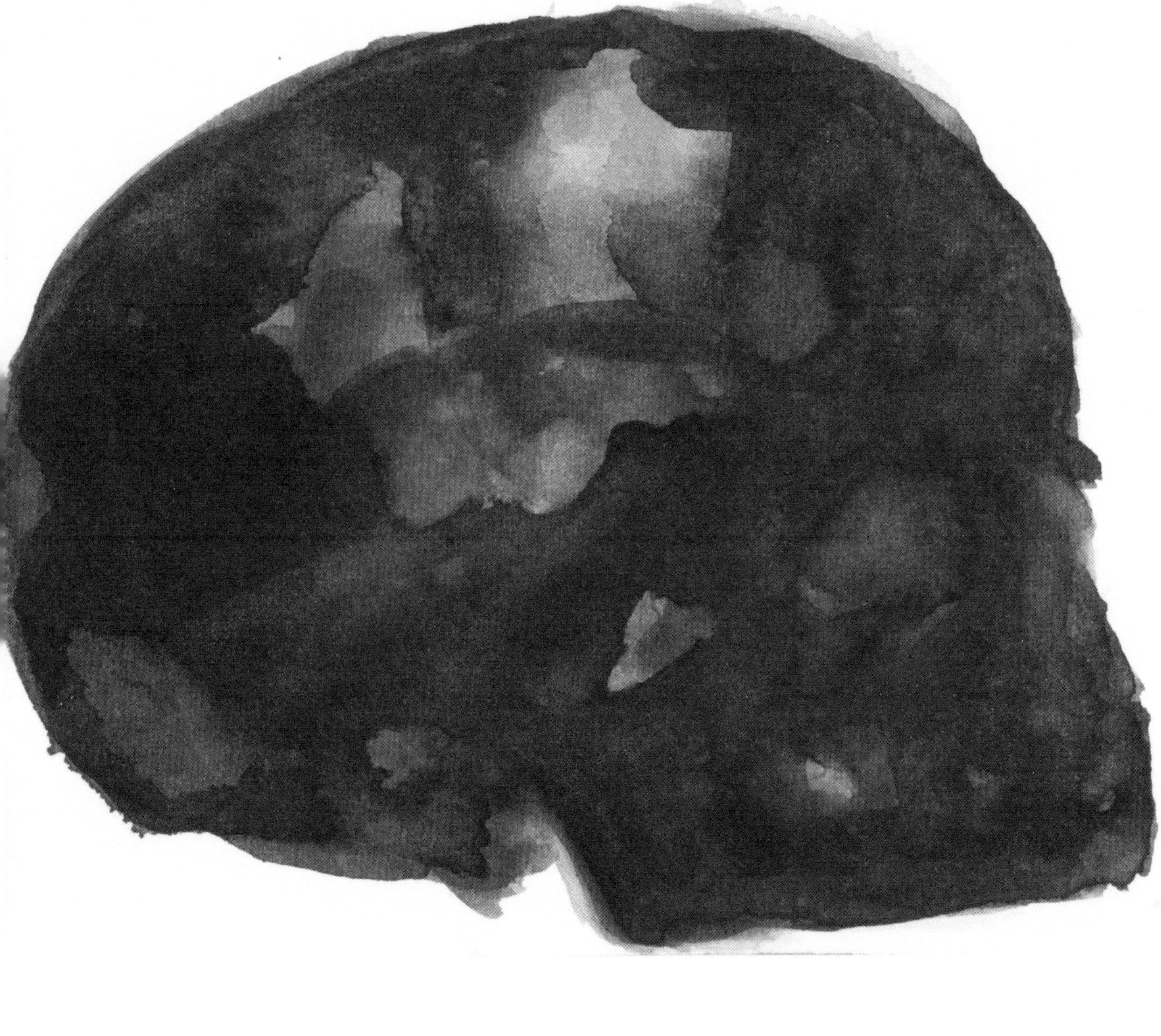

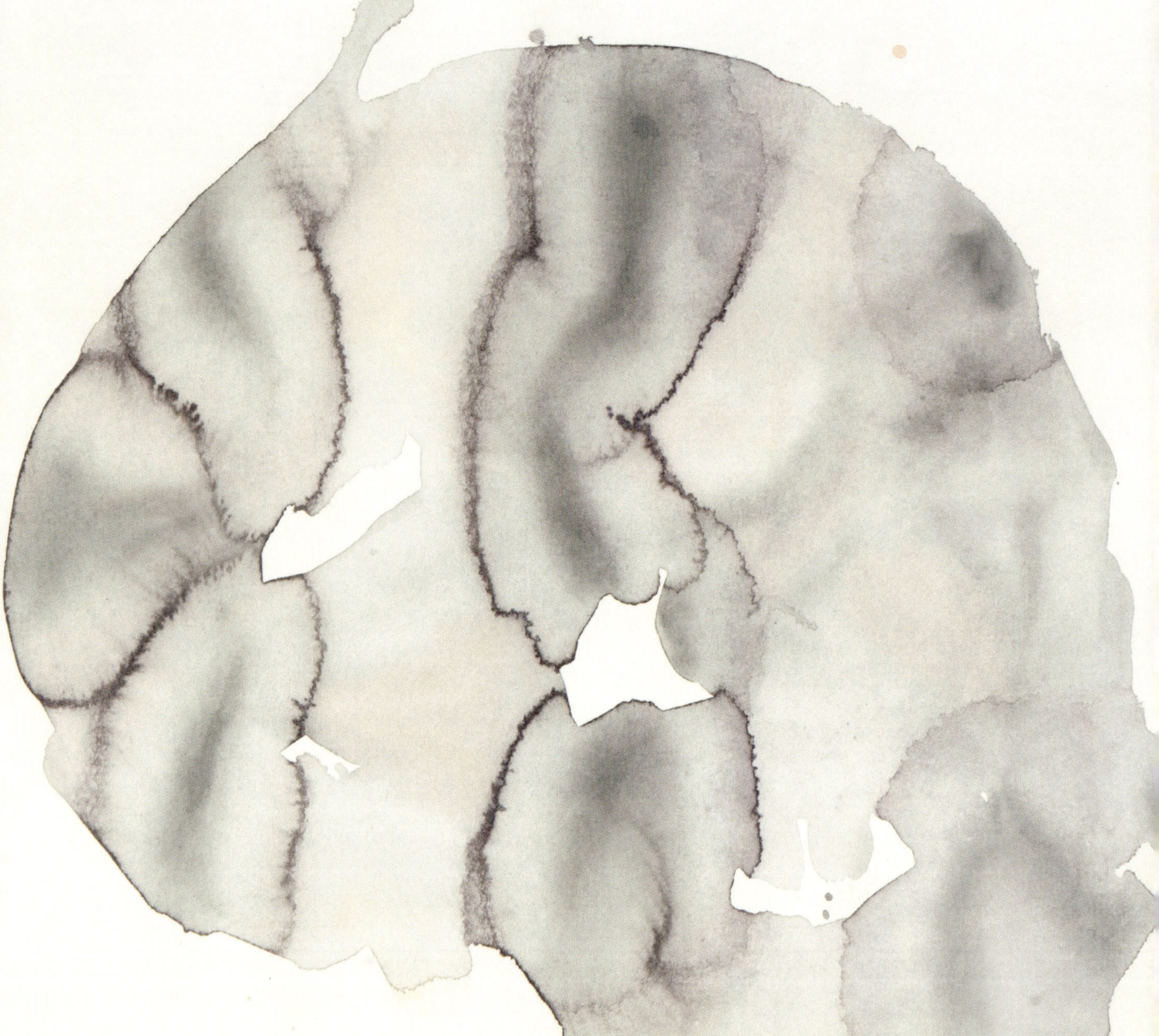

> The repeat-action of making them may be akin to repeating/talking about a trauma so as to exorcise it, externalise it, separate from it, see it. In other ways, the activity embodies the unending and daily consciousness of our own vulnerability, exaggerated in a place like South Africa – or constantly present, rather than a background reminder or awareness of mortality and loss.

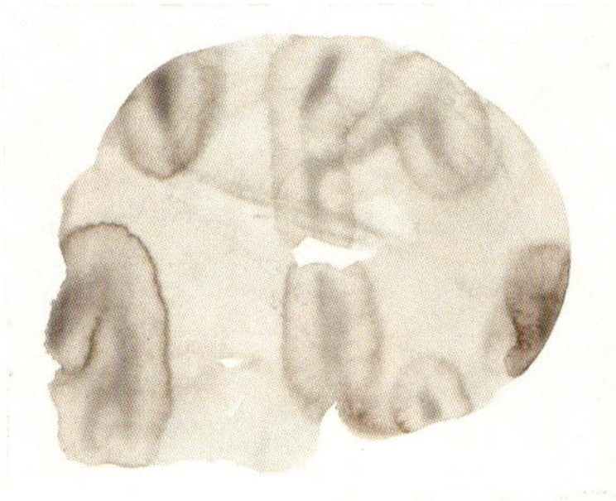

ABOVE: Joni Brenner, from *Wall of skulls*, watercolour on paper, 32 x 41 cm, 2008.

Brenner has remarked that engaging repeatedly and over a long period of time with the skulls has been paired with a wondering about the lived existence of those whose materiality has been reduced to bone. Brenner observes that our engagement with others' lives – such as mine with Mrs Konile[9] – makes us re-see ourselves: 'It's the reason to put oneself in other places. To see or be outside of oneself allows one to see oneself afresh.'

This remark was not only about her own work. She was talking about the differences or overlaps between how scientists and artists see. 'The objective/subjective perceptions of scientific and artistic knowledge and the perceived differences in approach to interpreting is certainly a key theme of the project,' she has said. She has suggested that objectivity may be a weakness of scientists who keep their subjects at arm's length. I agree. As anthropological and psychological sciences regularly show, subjectivity is very often a strength, and, in contrast, an attitude of unreflective detachment can be a liability. However, I question whether it is only scientists who keep their subjects at arm's length; whether, that is, there is anything inherent in art that makes one readily close to one's subjects, and I have to disagree. There are times when it is necessary to walk away from one's subject in order to see it clearly, and perhaps more importantly, to see oneself more clearly; but there is no substitute for close-up intimate knowledge regardless of whether one is an artist or scientist.

Out of what existential hole does the need to see and know ourselves spring? That we are real, maybe? That we are alive? Perhaps the need to see ourselves communicates that our here-ness matters, even if only to ourselves. This self-doubt about our own reality is similar to the doubts we entertain about others, of course, the feeling that it is impossible to completely know another person, the intractable strangeness of others. Turned inward, this impossibility as part of

LEFT: Joni Brenner, from *Wall of skulls*, watercolour on paper, 32 x 41 cm, 2008.

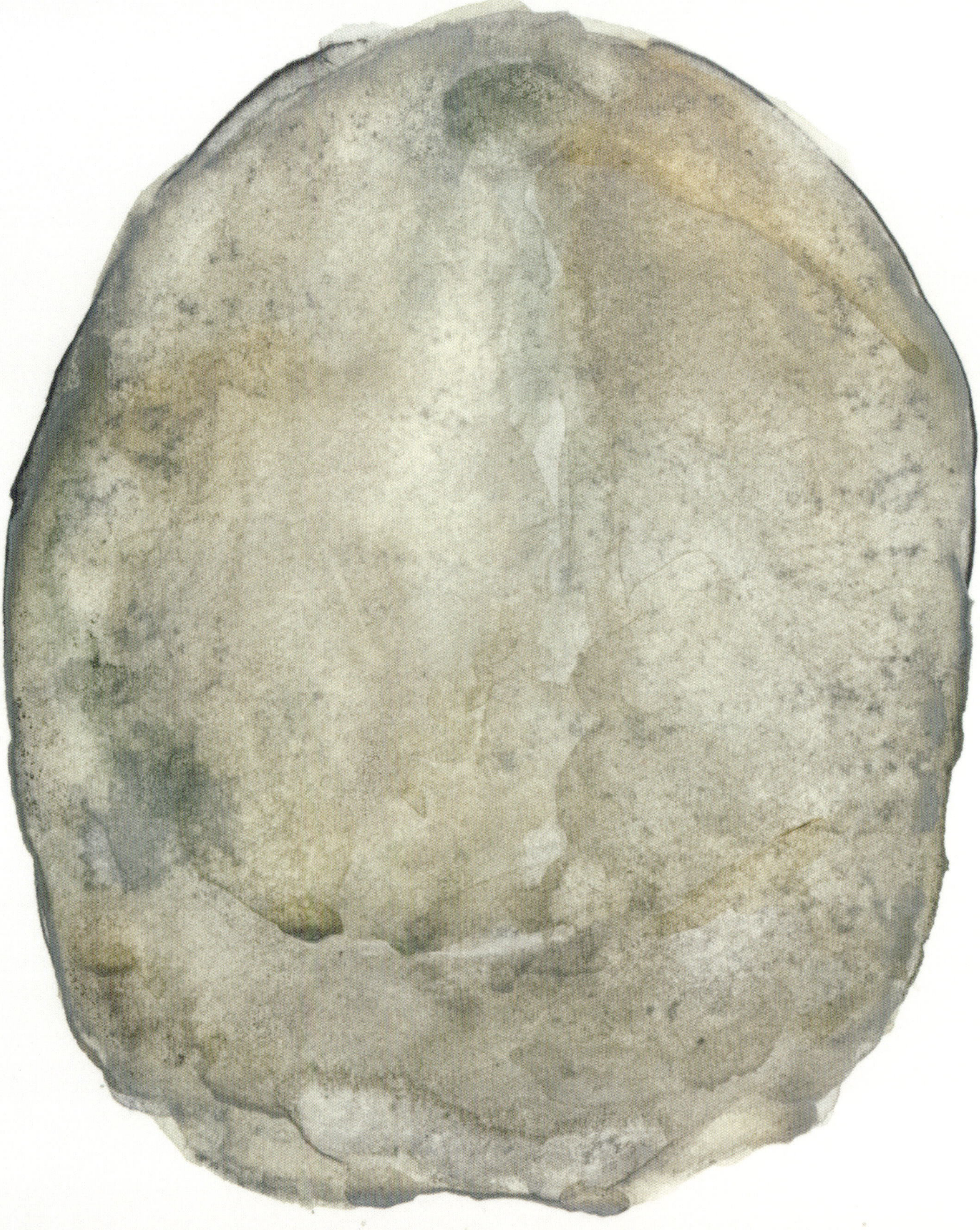

our existence is most lucid when we are being looked at, spoken to about ourselves, and we realise that how people identify us is replete with moments of misidentification. Even more troubling, perhaps, are those parts of ourselves that refuse knowing by ourselves, that keep slipping away from a direct gaze.

An impression may have been created that knowledge is an answer to uncertainty. If doubt is unsettling, scientific truth, to be sure, does not necessarily bring resolution. There are enough times when, even when convinced of the science behind findings, our knowing leaves behind more unhappiness than there otherwise would be. We know too well that representations are often forms of violence. There is an unavoidable politics to knowledge. Wherever you come across what is accepted as the truth, there you will find the workings of power, as we have learned from Berger, Said, Foucault, among others.

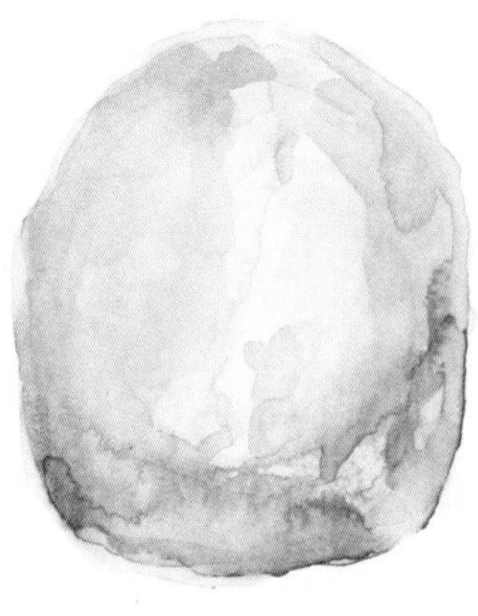

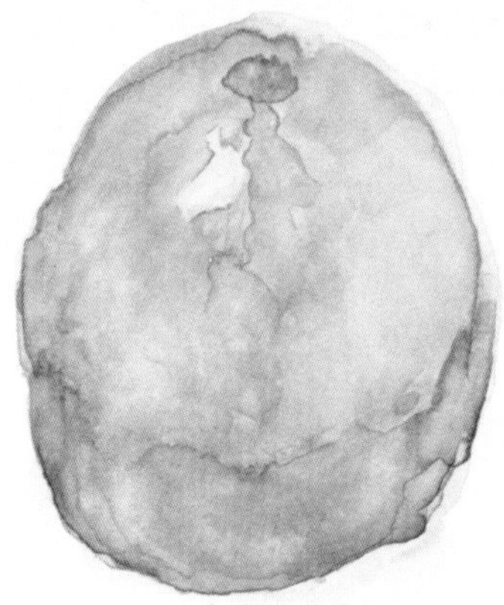

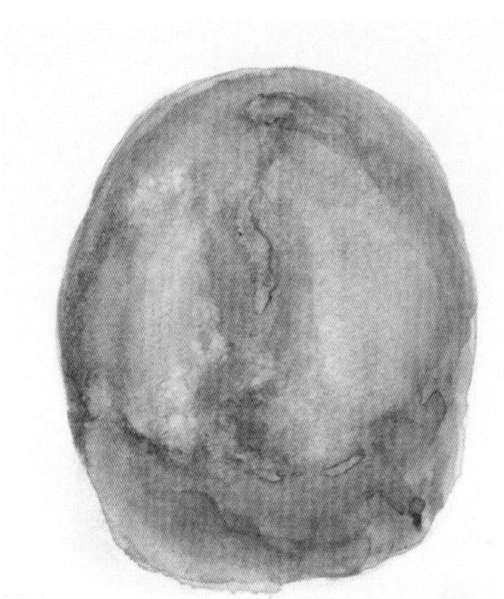

To return to the import of bones, when the remains of Zinakile Mkaba, Vuyisile Mini and Wilson Khayingo were about to be exhumed and returned to their families, a high-ranking office-bearer of the ANC was quoted as having said, 'The families won't be able to rest in peace until they know where the bones are.'[10] The three had been hanged for murder and sabotage at Pretoria Central prison on November 6, 1964, and their impending exhumation followed a change of policy that had declared the bodies of executed prisoners state property. The ANC official, Mathews Phosa, is said to have 'stressed the importance of families being able to bury their loved ones themselves, especially where this was a cultural prerequisite'.[11] Phosa is also said to have stated that 'you can't heal or reconcile on a lack of knowledge'.[12]

Of course one can. It is done on a daily basis. In fact, many a time some knowledge is an impediment to healing and reconciliation. Often enough, it is better not to know the graphic details. Yet something of exceeding interest is in that last paragraph. Here we learn that knowing where the bones of our dead are will not only bring peace and reconciliation to those who remain behind, but it is an imperative of some cultures for families to bury their dead. This cultural argument is not completely without foundation. We do need to know what we have lost for that loss to become part of our cultural past. The world is changed by what it loses as much as by what it gains. It is also true that some losses are

PAGE 82: Joni Brenner, from *Wall of skulls*, watercolour on paper, 21 x 15 cm, 2009.

PAGE 83 TOP: Joni Brenner, from *Wall of skulls*, watercolour on paper, 17.5 x 25 cm, 2009.

PAGE 83 CENTRE: Joni Brenner, from *Wall of skulls*, watercolour on paper, 17 x 25 cm, 2009.

PAGE 83 BOTTOM: Joni Brenner, from *Wall of skulls*, watercolour on paper, 17.5 x 25 cm, 2009.

in fact gains, such as having to lose childhood innocence on the way to understanding the world. On this theme of loss and its necessity in society, Brenner used Chimamanda Ngozi Adichie's phrase 'the world was silent when we died'[13] for one of her works, completed after the death of her long-time sitter, Wilson Mootane. It evokes for her, on the one hand, the tremendous human loss and pain that goes unacknowledged; and on the other hand, the significant way in which the world is altered or affected by these same losses.

But skulls or remains can tell only part of a story. Bones are mute. They are nevertheless suggestive of much. For some scientists and artists and cultures, bones generate more excitement than live bodies do. To become part of a culture, discipline or project, bones need interpreters – palaeontologists, painters, sculptors, kin. Stories must be told about them. They must be talked about, lectured on, explained, worshipped, searched for, retrieved, commemorated, archived, drawn, photographed and represented to restore their meaning. Knowledge must be built around them. Stories about loss and pain and discovery and recovery need to be constructed around them. Stories give flesh to the bare bones. Out of stories, we make culture, not from the bones of the dead, though the bones are the rationale for stories being told. Whereas in art, this impulse is clearer, science too is about telling certain stories. It is out of stories that we make society. Out of stories an individual constructs a self. Stories enable us to be identified as religious men or women, scientists, or artists, and of course, as mothers or sons, comrades or foes.

It turns out that stories are what settle us when uncertainty rises to trouble the day. In the same way, stories help us deal with too much data. When we want the truth but, naturally, can't know everything; or better, when we do know as much as we can but can't handle the truth, we'll settle for a plausible story.

Notes

1 Jansen, J. 2009. Knowledge in the Blood. Cape Town: UCT Press. p. 171.

2 Nel, K. 2009. "Disrupted knowledge" in *Penelope and the Cosmos*. Johannesburg: Circa on Jellicoe. p. 12.

3 Republic of South Africa 1995. Promotion of National Unity and Reconciliation Act, no 34 of 1995. Cape Town. Accessed at http://www.justice.gov.za/legislation/acts/1995-034.pdf

4 Truth and Reconciliation Commission 2003. Truth and Reconciliation Commission of South Africa Report. p. 350. The report can be accessed online at http://www.justice.gov.za/trc/report/index.htm

5 Truth and Reconciliation Commission 2003. Truth and Reconciliation Commission of South Africa Report. p. 428. The report can be accessed online at http://www.justice.gov.za/trc/report/index.htm

6 Truth and Reconciliation Commission 2003. Truth and Reconciliation Commission of South Africa Report. p. 8. The report can be accessed online at http://www.justice.gov.za/trc/report/index.htm

7 http://www.polity.org.za/polity/govdocs/commissions/1998/trc/3chap6.htm (see section on deaths in detention).

8 ibid.

9 The TRC testimony of Mrs Konile formed the subject of a book, *There was this goat* (2009), in which Antjie Krog, Nozisi Mpolweni and I strove to understand the apparently unintelligible account she gave of her experience of the loss of her son.

10 Accessed online at http://www.justice.gov.za/trc/media/1998/9804/s980407a.htm

11 ibid.

12 ibid.

13 Ngozi Adichie, C. 2006. *Half of a yellow sun*. USA: Alfred A. Knopf, Random House. p. 80.

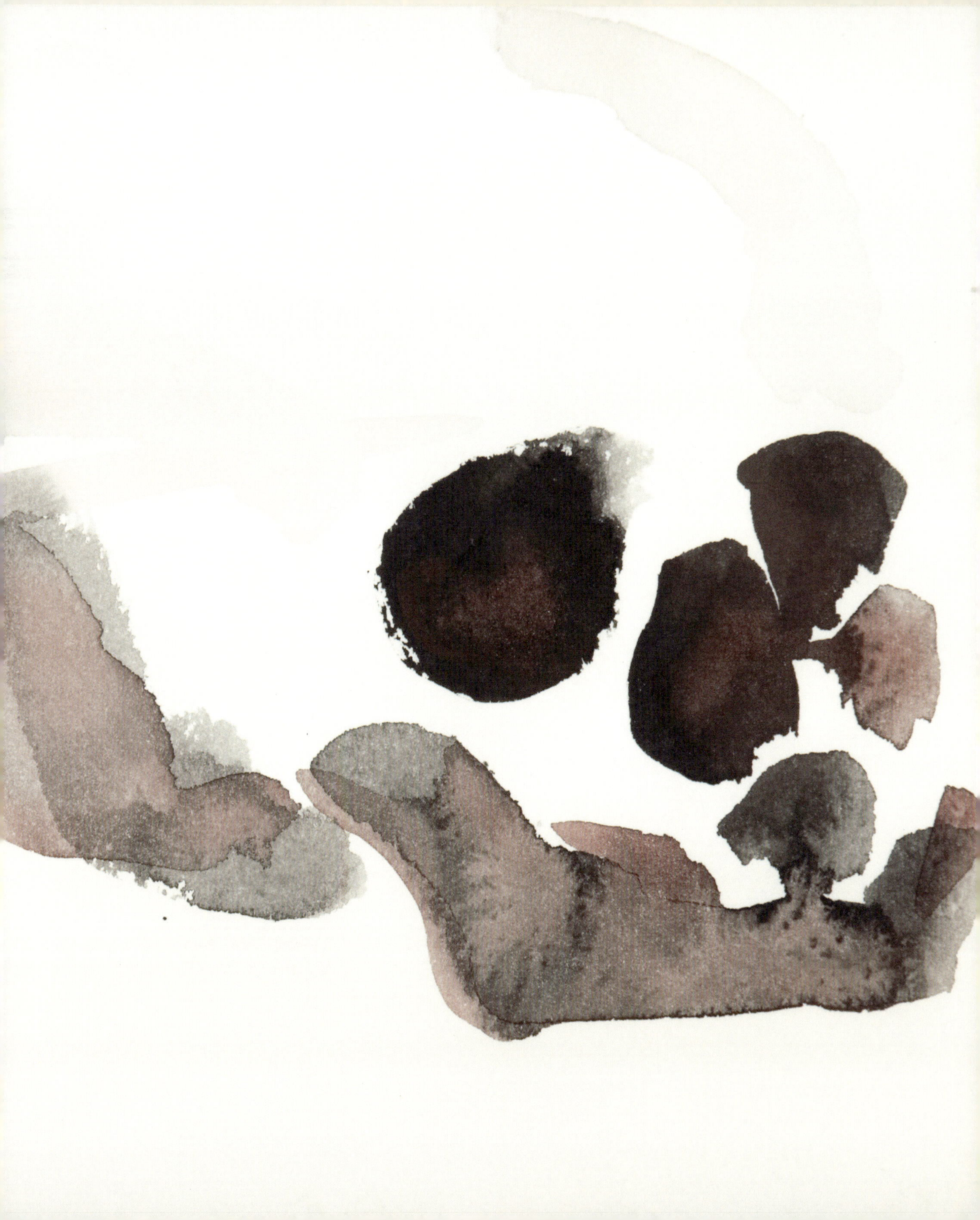

Chapter 5

Of words and skulls: Joni Brenner

Elizabeth Burroughs

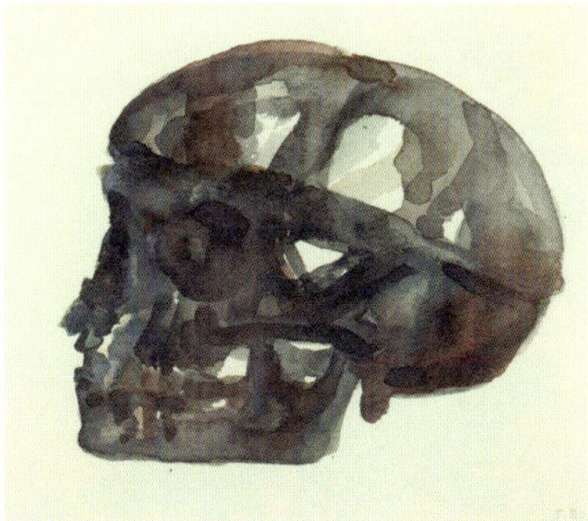

The props list for Act V Scene1 in *Hamlet* calls for not one, but three skulls. It was clearly less of a problem for the property master in the autumn of 1602, when the tragedy was first staged at the Globe, to obtain and display human tissue than it is now.

When Richard Burbage, the very first Hamlet, dressed in sombre black, raised the first skull from the gravedigger's heap, he considered who the person might have been – a fine lady whose breeding has meant nothing in the face of death; the second, a remarkable lawyer perhaps – 'a great buyer of land, with his statutes, his recognizances, his fines, his double vouchers, his recoveries' whose end is to have 'his fine pate full of fine dirt'. The third skull, however, the grave-digger identifies as the king's jester's skull, that of Yorick, more than two decades dead. This news electrifies Hamlet, who had known him well; indeed, as a child, he had ridden on this man's back 'a thousand times'. Hamlet's exposition on the inexorability of death, its reductive nature of all that is great in a human, whether Caesar or Alexander, forms the prologue for all the deaths around Ophelia's grave that are to follow.

In Joni's studio, three skulls on her bench form a riveting nucleus for everything else that goes on around them. She may not be able to identify one of the three as Yorick, though the one – not a real skull, but a cast this time – we all know

LEFT: Joni Brenner, *Revelation series,* watercolour on paper, 15 x 21 cm, 2005.

ABOVE: Joni Brenner, *Revelation series,* watercolour on paper, 18 x 25 cm, 2005.

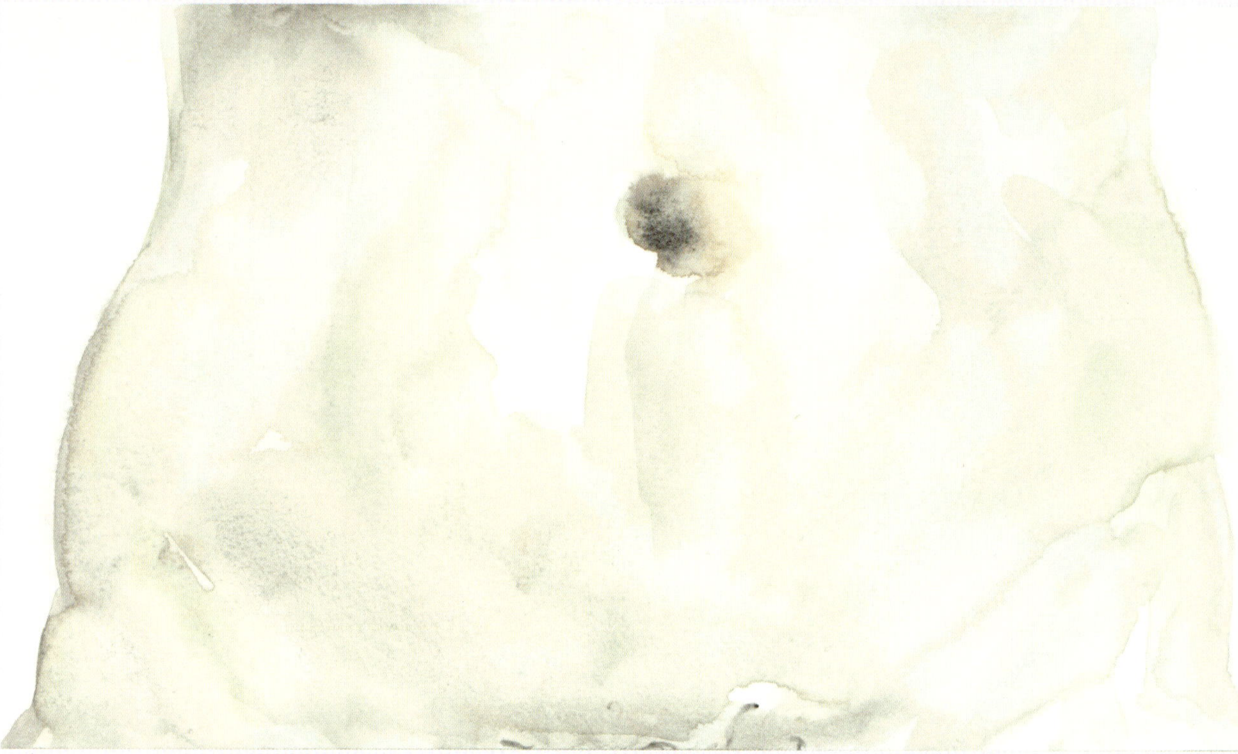

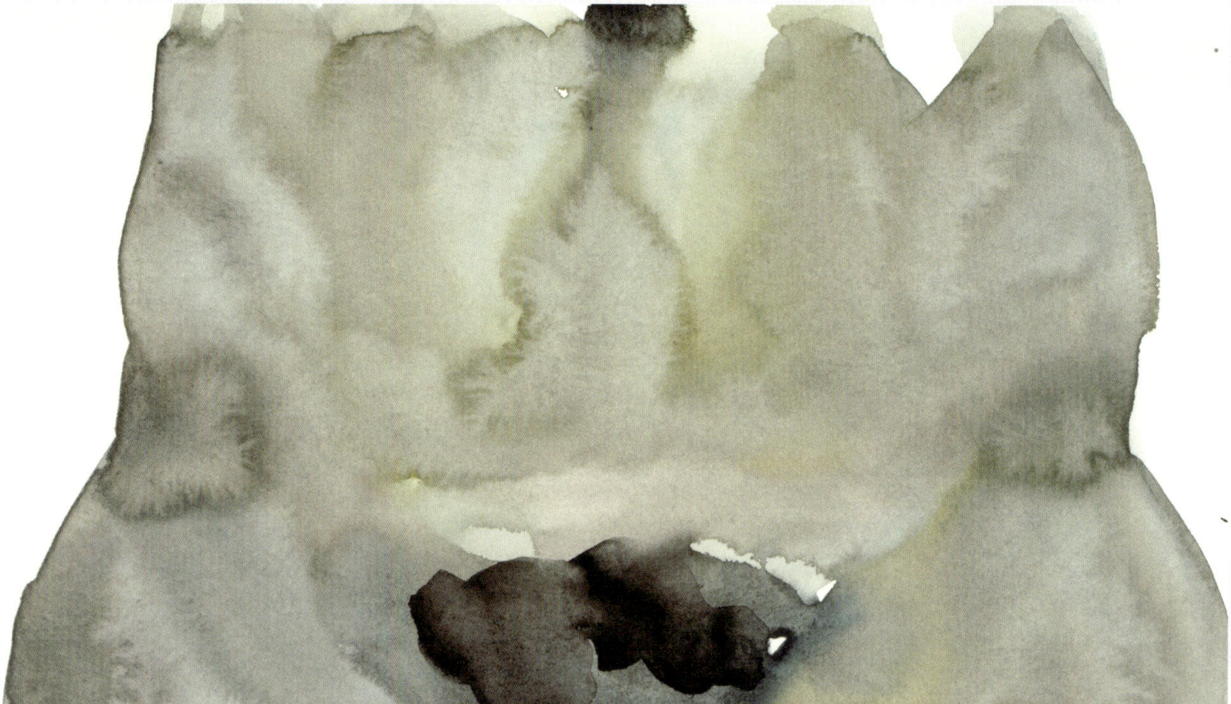

as the Taung child. These three presences are simultaneously anonymous but also deeply, intimately familiar, for they have been the source of ongoing meditations in watercolour, a focused calligraphy on these most human of forms.

Joni's friend, Lynne Slonimsky, has written a sequence of haikus, which, in their sparseness, form a kind of objective correlative for the making of these works and for the images themselves:

Through watercolours
élan vital is restored
no longer dry bones

Day by day by day
focusing on presences
no more emptiness

The works, known collectively when they're talked about as 'the skulls', all small, all immediate, have been done over a period of five years and form a formidable record of intimate observation. Here, Joni renders the curve of the cranium with a sweep of water tinctured just a little; the cheekbone with a single mark warmed with a hint of red within the grey; lustrous black swept swiftly, lightly into the eye sockets and the wedge of the nasal cavity. The delicate image has the grace of a moment's thought, and is, but it is also the culmination of hundreds of such fingering gazes, until the distance between the object and the maker has completely collapsed: Joni even painted these loved skulls from memory during her stay in Paris.

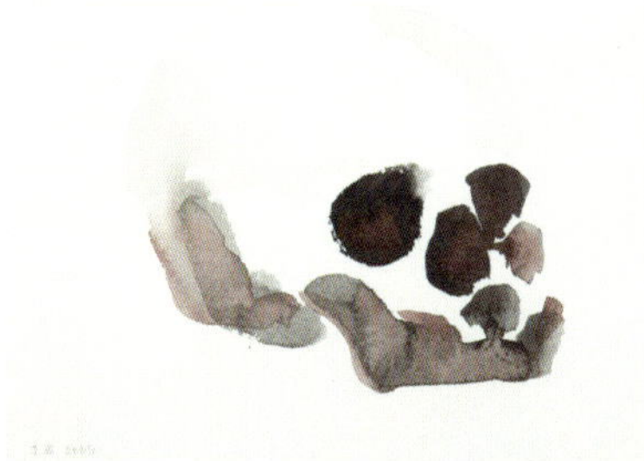

Joni Brenner, *Revelation series*, watercolour on paper, 15 x 21 cm, 2005.

But not all of the skull paintings are like that. Some feel feverish, as if she were racing against time, against the constraint of the watery medium, against the protean nature of the skull's appearance. Against the threatening internal chaos, which can only be managed by speed and grace, like a skater who moves so fast that she is falling all the time, but saved from falling by moving so fast. Against the demands on her time of teaching Renaissance portraiture or African photography, of being a daughter needing to sell a house, of being in a relationship where the possibility of becoming parents to a child is real.

LEFT ABOVE: Joni Brenner, from *Navel:Paris*, watercolour on paper, 19 x 33 cm, 2010.

LEFT BELOW Joni Brenner, from *Navel:Paris*, watercolour on paper, 19 x 33 cm, 2010.

Joni Brenner, from *Taung series*, watercolour on paper, 25 x 35.5 cm, 2010.

The skull paintings are much less anatomical renderings, though clearly they are that too. Each is an identifiable portrait of one of the skulls, and the visitor to the studio will always know which. Even more, perhaps, the watercolours are a diary of the observer, the maker: how she sees deeply affects what she sees, and how she sees is deeply affected by how she is in the world at the moment that she selects the skull she will look at, the paper she will use, the blocks of pigment she will use ... at that time of the morning, or at that time of the afternoon when the light slants in from the west. This sheet of paper is part of the precious stock bought in Paris, and this little cube of Old Holland Violet-grey, almost finished now, was from the trip before last to New York. When the painting's done, she has a sense, though not foregrounded, of the warm lentil and goat's milk cheese salad she will make for her and Scott over another glass of the Merlot he opened last night. And through it all, like a dull bass-line, that melancholic distress that she still hasn't shaken after her stay at the Cité, of living in a city without museums.

They talk over the fragrant food about why contextualised subjectivity is regarded as being an acceptable element of artistic thought, but which somehow is or must be excised in the exercise of scientific enquiry, or at least in its formal representation. She reads Scott a quotation from Malcolm Gladwell that I'd sent. Gladwell argues that 'who we are cannot be separated from where we're from', and, Joni tells Scott that I think Gladwell should have added '*when* we're from' as well: how inconvenient it was, not to say presumptuous, to have an Australian upstart declaring that a tiny skull, blasted out of a lime-works in a godforsakenly remote place called Taung, represented an early ancestral forerunner to *Homo sapiens*. Certainly, it was much easier to turn a unified European scientific back on the southern African fossil than have it re-arrange the mental family tree. So too, in the past few years, the evidence at Çatalhöyök has been re-evaluated, and James Mellaert's mid-1960s account of it as a matriarchal society poised between nomadism and a settled agricultural existence seems to owe more to the powerful feminist discourses current while he was excavating and writing than it did to much of the hard-and-fast material evidence emerging from the site. June Singer, a Jungian analyst, in her *Boundaries of the soul*, is unafraid to review Jung's view of women, and, in a subsequent revision of her own book, to re-evaluate her earlier

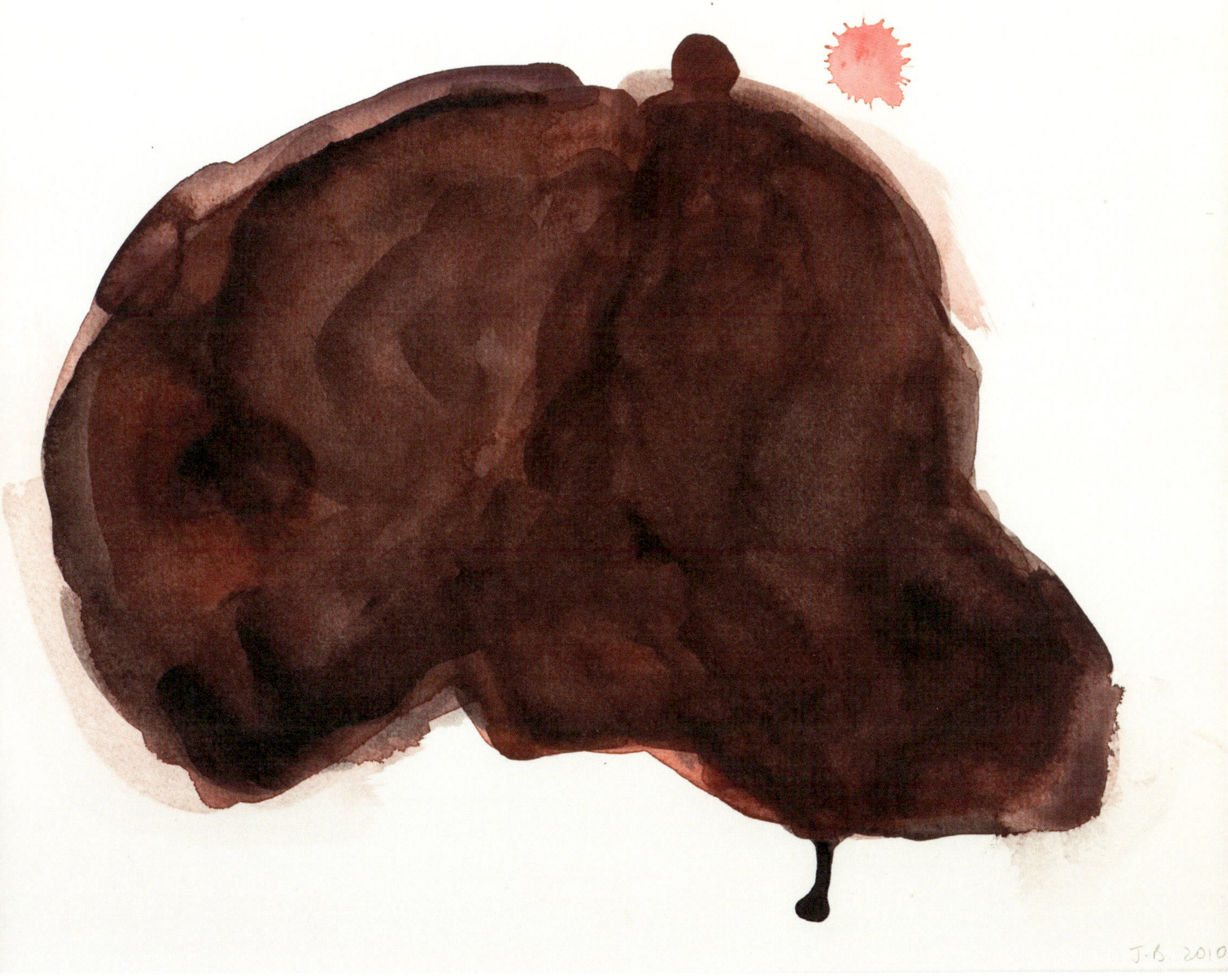
J.B. 2010

perspective. As Scott and Joni wash the dishes, she wonders where the notion of knowledge as a static and relatively unchanging body of knowledge seems to have taken root. Scott says the new rhetoric about societies needing to be learning societies comes from a recognition of the profoundly changed nature of knowledge, but that for many, the notion is really no more than a catchy slogan.

Looking through the wealth of unframed skulls with Joni, I know that the skull she views is arguably the same skull as it was the day before, a 'fact', if you like, but Joni is not the same. Her knowledge base is not the same: she has been to the funeral of a much-loved colleague and friend – one, it seems, in a series of losses that have come thick and fast recently; has read James Lord's biography of Giacometti; has had an altercation and not yet made up; has had a joyful, life-enhancing photograph taken of herself by Malik Sidibé in his Bamako studio with the classic striped backdrop, a gift for herself and for Scott. Feelings, ideas, emotions, loss and pleasure are the loam that nurture the next painting, and the next. Joni has spoken a lot about Giacometti. She has found resonance in the fact that his work seems to have been driven by his sense of human frailty and the 'fantastic energy' it requires for people to continue to be. She understands feelingly that he was driven by the belief that any effort to capture what he saw was doomed to failure in any case; and, perhaps, even worse, that success would mean the task was done and there would be nothing more to do. His work was not about the final object, as Lord's series of photographs of the portrait Giacometti did of him so clearly show – it was the process, the pursuit of the vision that was the life-sustaining effort.

While Joni clearly identifies with something in Giacometti's approach, in the focused – is it obsessive? – re-iteration of the subject, her effort is focused on understanding what is, and is not present, in the skulls. There is so much that is unknown and unknowable, she says. Every effort at representation is a probe, a search for the eidetic truth, even while each painting disconfirms the possibility of an absolute knowing. The similarity between this form of poetic, visual enquiry and the search for scientific answers to the questions about, say, the genetic origin of the species, or why it has developed the capacity to take pleasure in working things out, is perhaps nothing less than this repeated and manifold return to

Malick Sidibé, *portrait of Joni Brenner*, photograph, 22.5 x 16.5 cm, 2009.

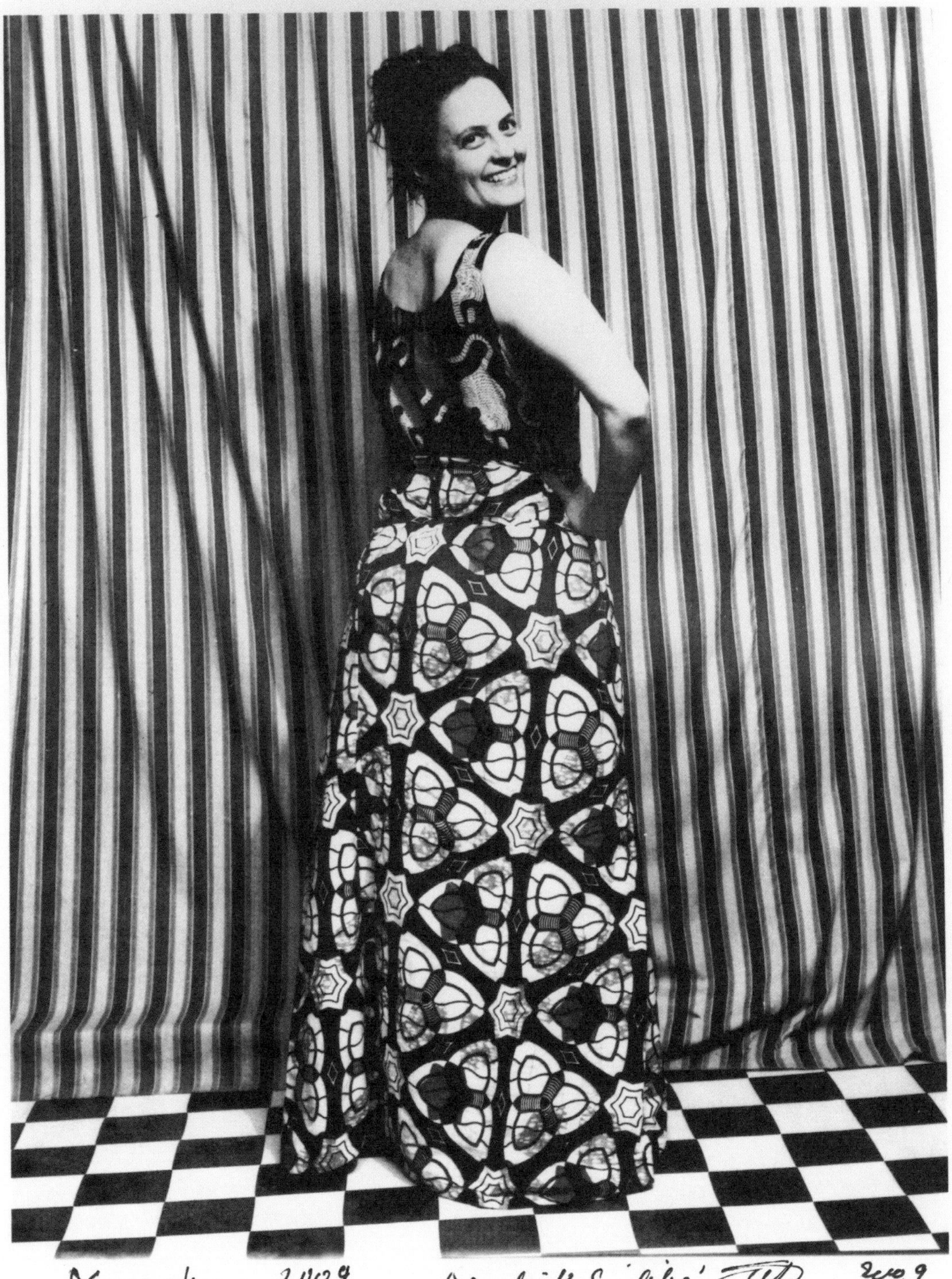

Novembre - 2009 Malick Sidibé 2009

the same issue, looking for an answer or answers that approximate most satisfactorily to what is perceived to be out there.

Here in this moment
Temporary suspension
Before it passes

Such silent repose
Watching breath rising
and falling
Exquisite balance

Each moment that I
Focus on what is present
Heals the emptiness

Day by day by day
Before the look of the other
A being transformed

The idea of having an exhibition of skulls must have come during one of those moments when she looked at the accumulated images, each revealing something a little different. It was a thought that, once it had come, nudged repeatedly against the question of who this person was – who these people were whose skulls, through chance and circumstance, had passed into her keeping. Some friends shudder at their presence in the studio, asking why she doesn't dispose of them as decently as possible, but she has come to have great reverence for these mortal remains in her care, and no action seems more respectful than keeping them safe, observing them, seeking to understand something of the quintessential uniqueness of each. The cast of the Taung child's skull and brain came later than the two skulls, and it was an effort to train her eye and hand to the new contours, so similar, and yet so different to the ones she was used to. Respect for the other skulls has now spilled over into tenderness. Who was this child? What was the circumstance of his or her untimely death? What loss and seeking would there have been by distraught family? She knows, from having watched how two thrushes sought to protect their fledgling, which had fallen from the nest, that

Joni Brenner, from *Wall of skulls*, watercolour on paper, 25 x 35.5 cm, 2008.

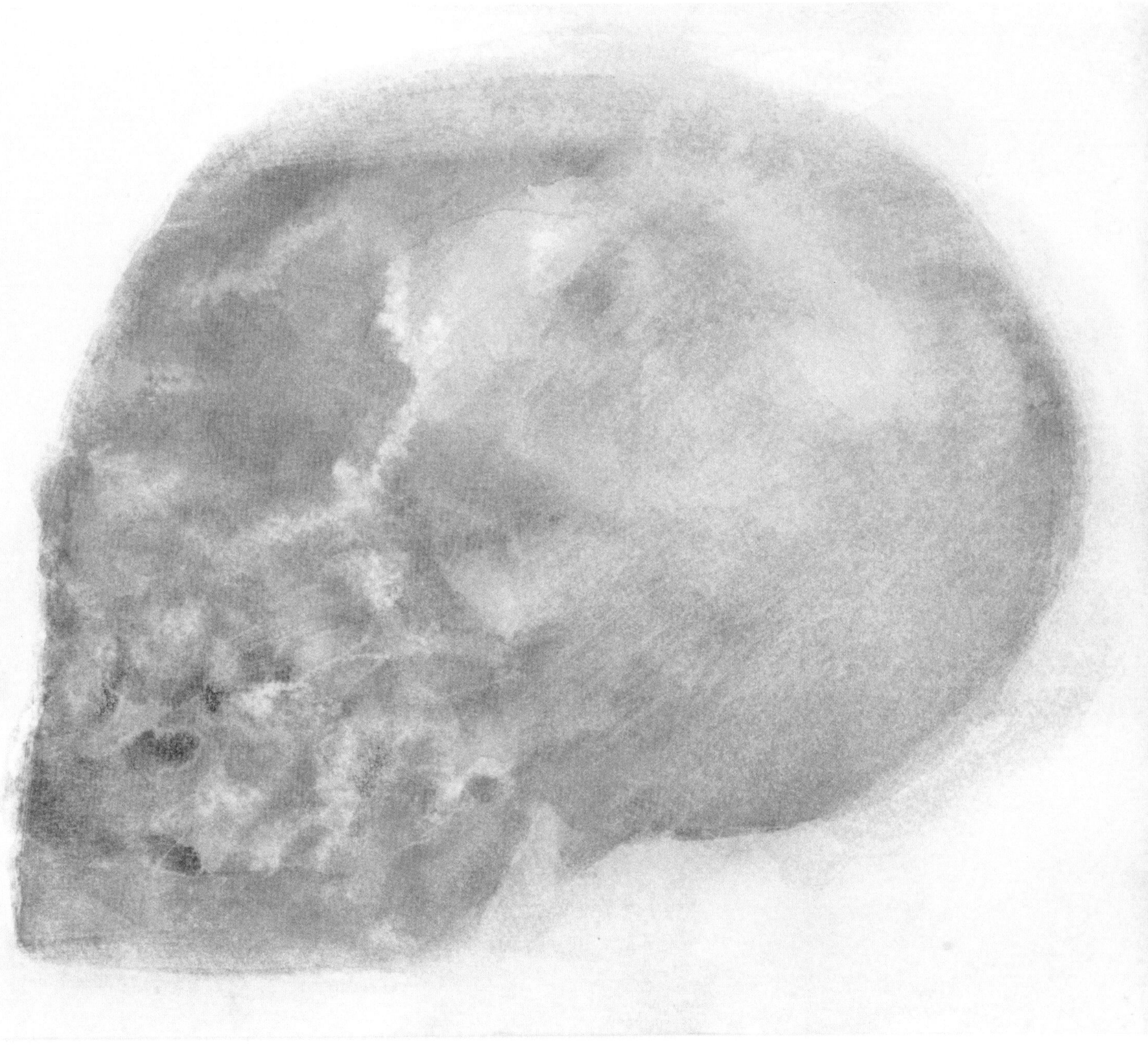

the mother of this child would have been distressed in the same deep, helpless way. Love is an instinctual thing. Somewhere she'd heard that the people in the doomed 9/11 planes had, as their last acts, texted their loved ones to tell them how much they were loved.

Love and death. In a recent piece that Joni wrote about the death of her long-time sitter and friend, Wilson Mootane, she quotes the critic Michel Leiris who said that 'there are moments that may be called crises and these are the only ones that count in life'. Joni is not one of those crazy-makers whose life is only worth living if there is drama in it, so it is interesting that she chose Leiris's quotation to help her make sense of Wilson's death, which happened at the beginning of 2010. She has written a lot about her work, about Wilson too. I have always sensed a kind of ambiguity in Joni's writing about her relationship with him. It was a relationship between a younger white woman and an older black man; being South Africans, she was the more privileged, able – albeit from a part-time university salary – to pay him for the time that he came to be her sitter. And because these were the demographic parameters of the relationship, it was perhaps difficult to put into words what its real significance was. What is a sitter to the artist? Wilson's regular Sunday visits to her studio provided the metronomic rhythm to her work, gave impetus when energy was low, provided the catalyst for works in a range of materials from wax and plasticine, to oils on canvas, jelutong, Supawood, granite and marble. While it was clear his presence was the *sine qua non* for her work, Joni's focus seemed always to be on the symbolic functions of portraiture, the tension between representation of the moment and the effluxion of time, the shadow between the desire to capture for always the reality of the living and inevitable death, the contradiction that the momentary is static and can only ever be suggestive of the fugitive whole. Wilson would sit peacefully for hours while she worked feverishly, sometimes offering her words of encouragement or comfort. Sometimes, he would prepare the clay she would work with. His presence was steadfast. What Joni did not really understand was how much her work, abstract as it is, was a record of a living, long-standing relationship. The seventeen years of companionable silence while she created and Wilson bore witness to the work she did functioned in contradistinction to all

Wilson Mootane in Brenner's studio, Johannesburg. Photograph by Joni Brenner, 2009.

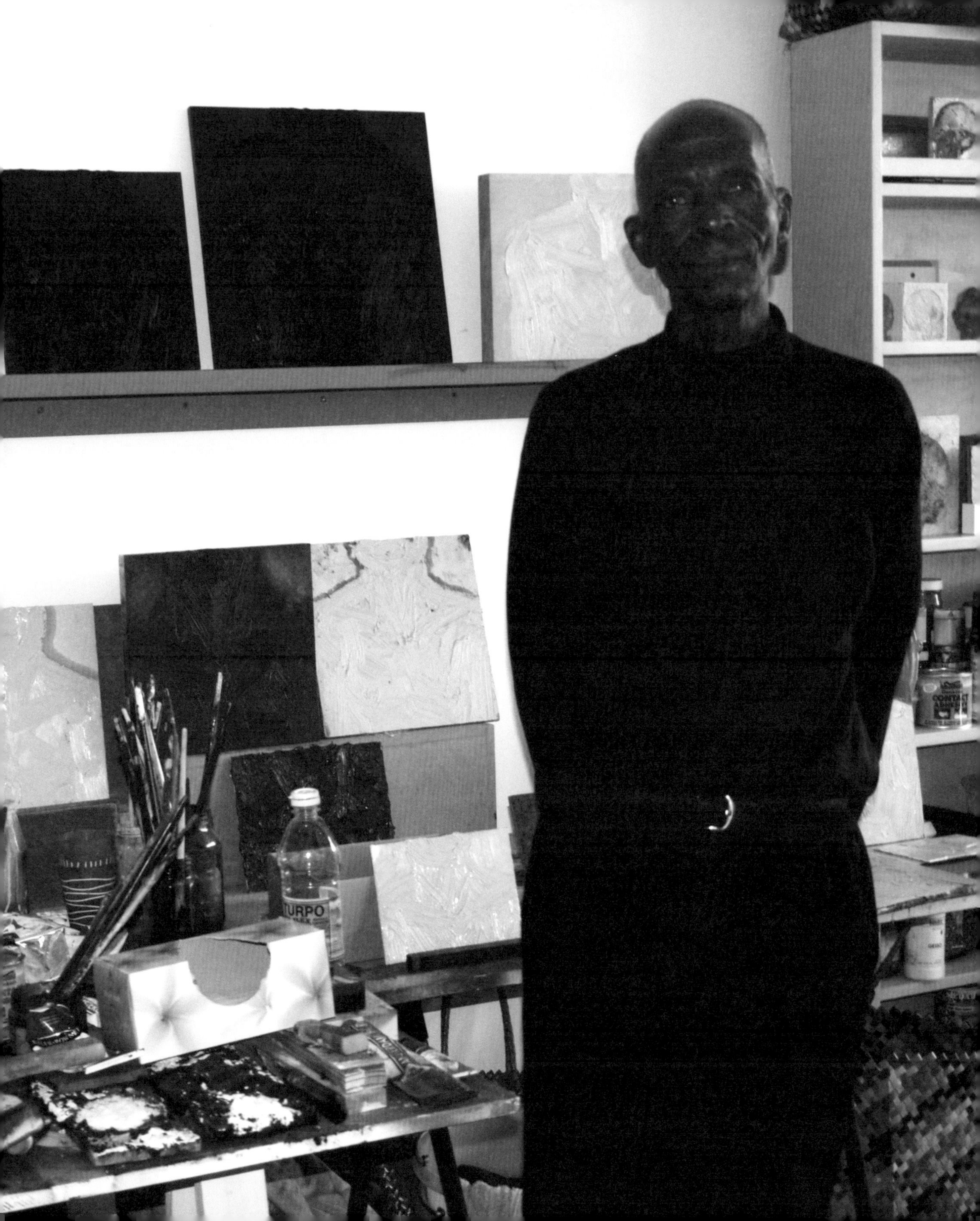
TURPO
CONTACT

the intellectual conundrums that her passion for portraiture occasioned. Last year though, Wilson's health began to falter, and the phone calls and emails from that time reflected Joni's fears.

Wilson's death has been one of those times of crisis that really count. Everything that went before, and everything that comes after, will not be the same because, as things worked out, he died quietly in her arms, giving a retrospective depth and value to all that went before. The two pieces that Joni wrote tell the story so eloquently that it is not necessary to tell it again here, but I have alluded to it, because it is perhaps one of the most important things that has happened during the time that this exhibition and book have been gestating. It is by no means the only one. Joni and Karel and I have spoken time and again about the life and death of Annemarie, Karel's mother, and mine, and a mother, too, to Joni, though not of course in the biological sense; Joni and Scott have needed to find a way to be together; Joni's parents have moved countries; and she has moved from one apartment to another; she has also travelled to West Africa, England, France and the United States. These are not necessarily the milestones that appear on one's CV, as do the solo exhibitions and the representations on group shows, but they are often the wellsprings for growth and development.

Joni's trip to Paris, where she'd been awarded time at the Cité, in May last year, was not ideal in terms of the *Life of bone* project, and difficult coming as it did soon after Wilson's death, and yet, taking her out of her usual space, it provided a time of reflection and of new beginnings. Thrown back on her own resources, she began, for the first time in years, to be her own sitter. A wall of forearms, sensuous bellies, hands, faces, fists came back with her, some painted to a litany of the names of the Jewish dead of Paris which were read aloud in a memorial service over a period of days in a museum close to her apartment. At much the same time, she painted two breast-like images in memory of Louise Bourgeois' death, and we chuckled about her embroidered handkerchief, which reads, 'I've been to hell and back, and let me tell you, it was wonderful.'

The lives and the work of scientists, whether they are palaeoanthropologists, archaeologists or astronomers are just as deeply influenced by their own trips to hell and back, their own crises, and it is certain that these will influence how the

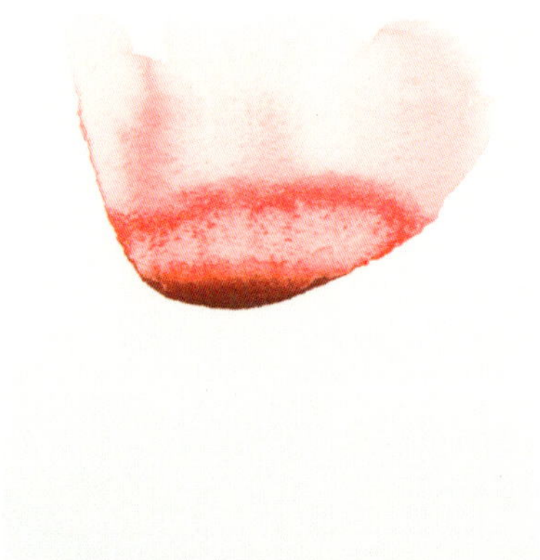

ABOVE: Joni Brenner, *Homage to Louise Bourgeois*, watercolour on paper, 10 x 15 cm, 2010.

RIGHT: Joni Brenner, *Homage to Louise Bourgeois*, watercolour on paper, 21 x 15 cm, 2010.

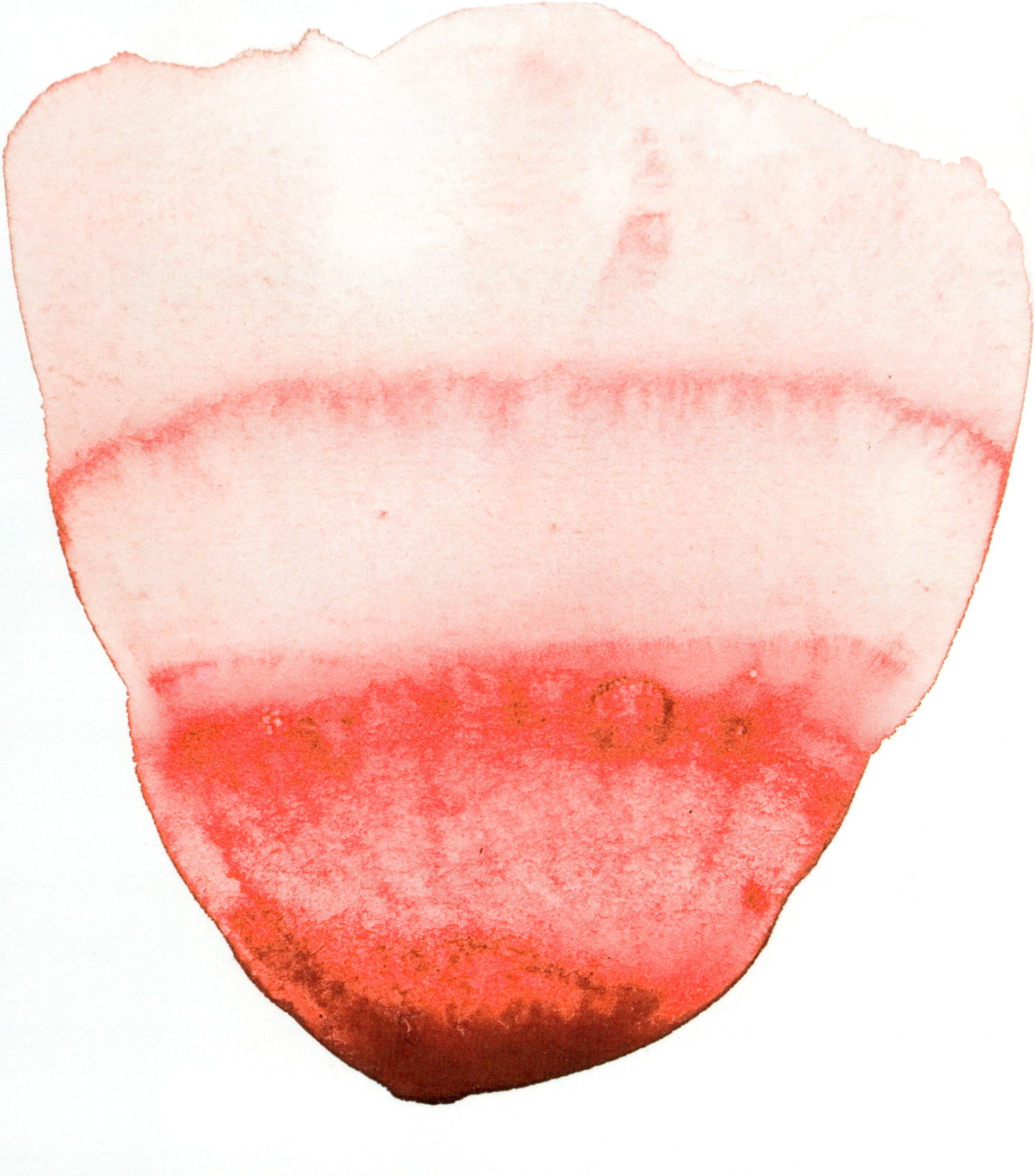

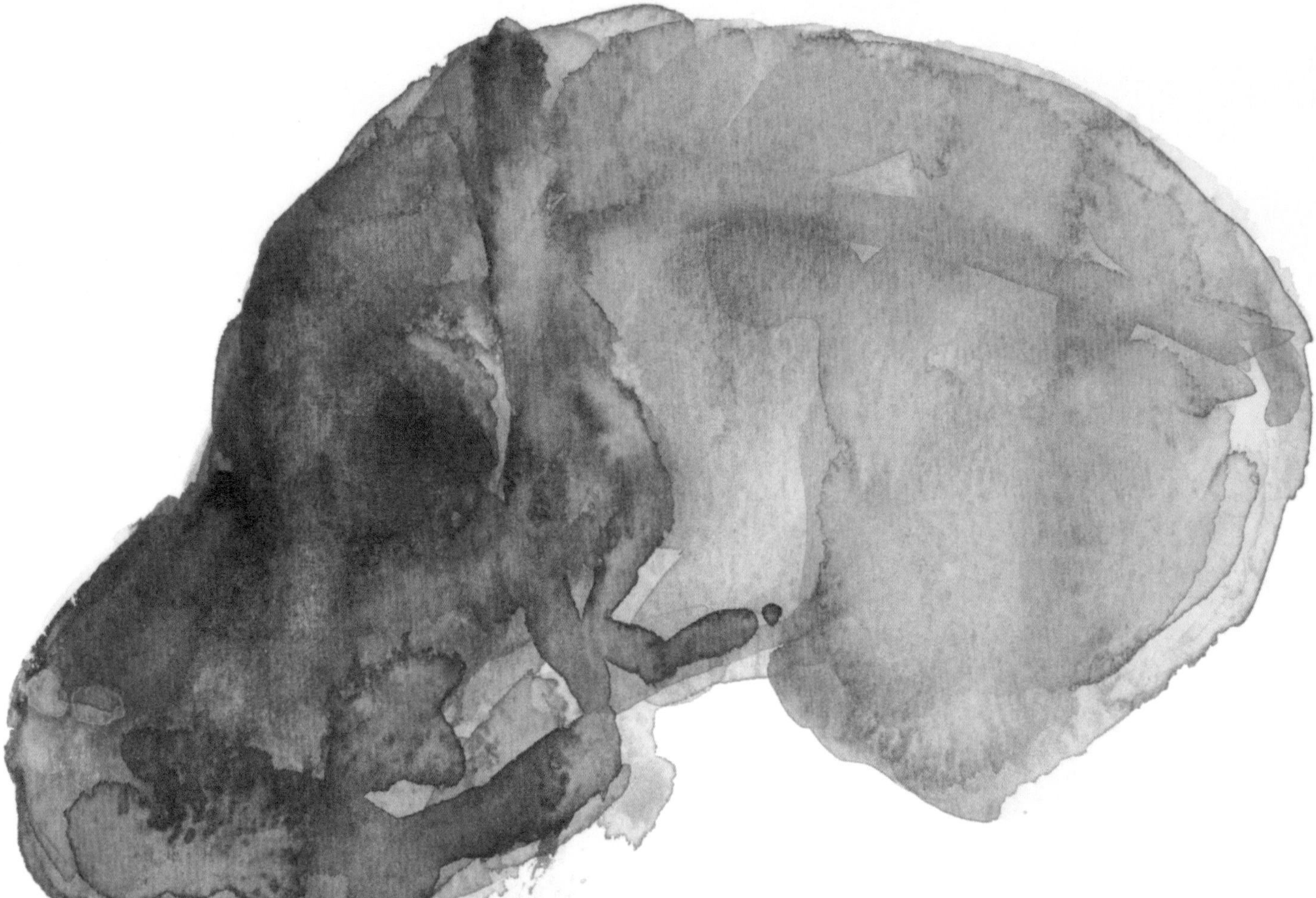

data is read. The texts, like Joni's skull series may not allude to the highs and lows that have driven the work forward, but they are nonetheless there. New data may provide the missing keystone in the theory, or make one wonder whether the structure is an arch after all. Every new hominid or hominin skull – or pelvis or set of metatarsals – constitutes one of those crises that really count in palaeoanthropology. Every new comparison dashes certain hypotheses, strengthens certain lines of argument, raises new sets of questions. Every scientific article is a deliberate weighing up of the possibilities, a creation of the most satisfactory solution to an incomplete puzzle, an attempt to know the unknowable.

Joni Brenner, from *Taung series*, watercolour on paper, 18 x 25.5 cm, 2010

During work on the project, Joni has commented repeatedly how the scientists have wished to express something of their understanding in a mode that is not strictly scientific and closer to the artistic: is it because there is an imaginative residue that is somehow denied by the accepted modes of expression the discipline allows? Is it, equally that, though a picture is proverbially worth a thousand words, the artists too have longed so ardently to supplement their usual non-lingual avenues of expression with the written word?

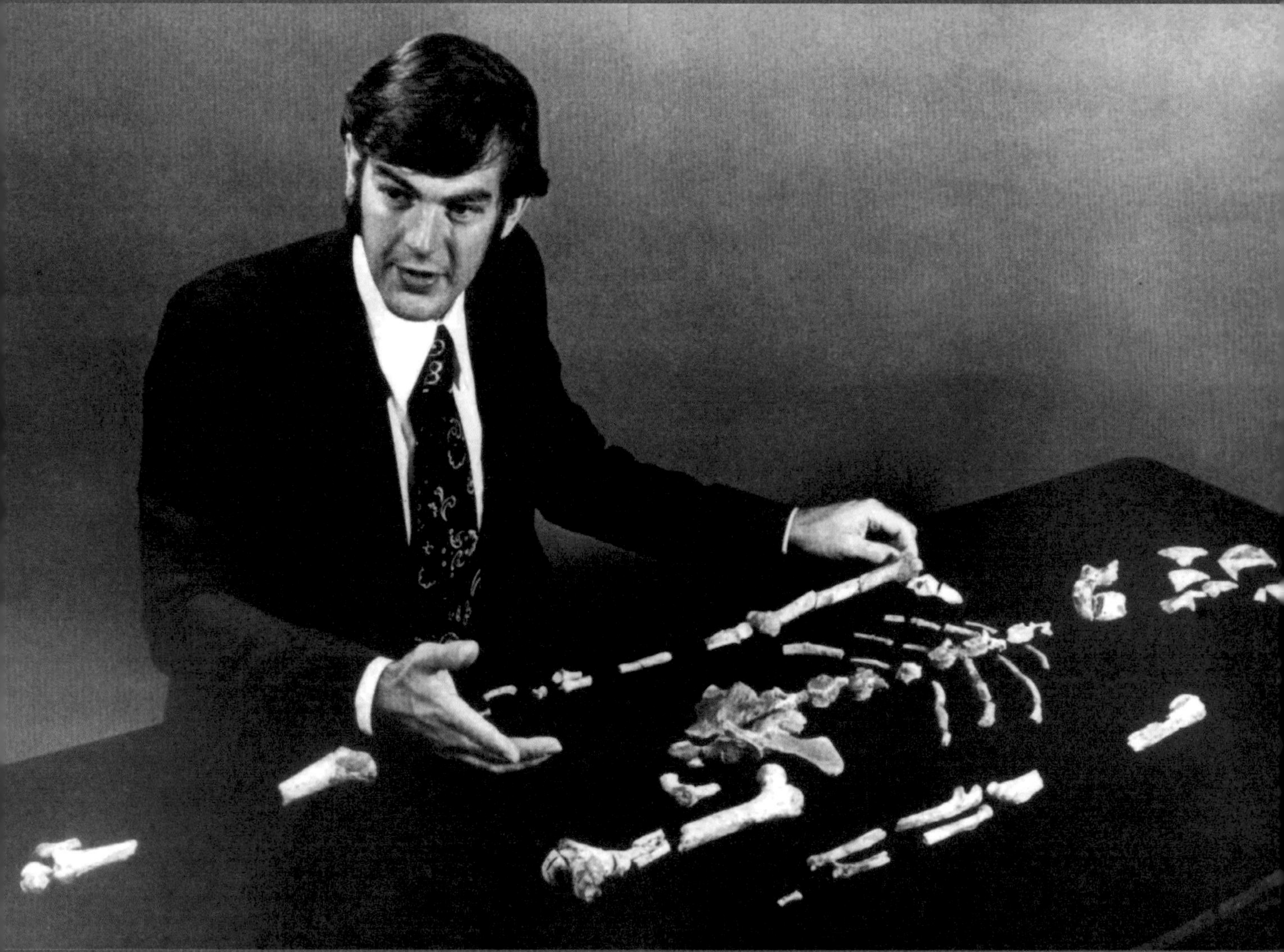

Chapter 6

Where do we come from? Who are we? Where are we going?[1]

Donald Johanson

Throughout the history of life on this planet untold millions of species have come and gone. Some, like the cockroach, haven't changed much since the early Cretaceous period. Others lost the competition for resources and went extinct, or were wiped out by a single cosmic cataclysm. Many underwent adaptive change in order to accommodate changes in their environment. One species in particular excelled – capitalising on new challenges that resulted in a larger brain, a better method of locomotion, and, eventually, the ability to significantly control its surroundings. With a population of more than 6.5 billion, *Homo sapiens* is by anyone's measure a wildly successful species whose domination of Earth is evident everywhere.

Five hundred thousand years ago, humans were able to make fire, flake stone tools, engage in organised hunting, and probably communicate using rudimentary language. But relatively recently, perhaps only 50,000 years ago, our direct ancestors underwent a dramatic behavioural change that distinguishes us from all other animals. Three-and-a-alf million years ago, one of man's earliest ancestors left footprints in volcanic ash at Laetoli, Tanzania; less than 50 years ago, a new kind of hominid left footprints on the moon. Compared to other humans, *sapiens* have only been around a short time. So what could have caused such a monumental leap?

I believe that human evolution is the product of a synergetic combination of biological and perhaps, more importantly, cultural evolution. Culture provides the magic of infinite innovation, and is singularly human.

Don Johanson and Lucy, 1975, courtesy of the Institute of Human Origins, Arizona State University.

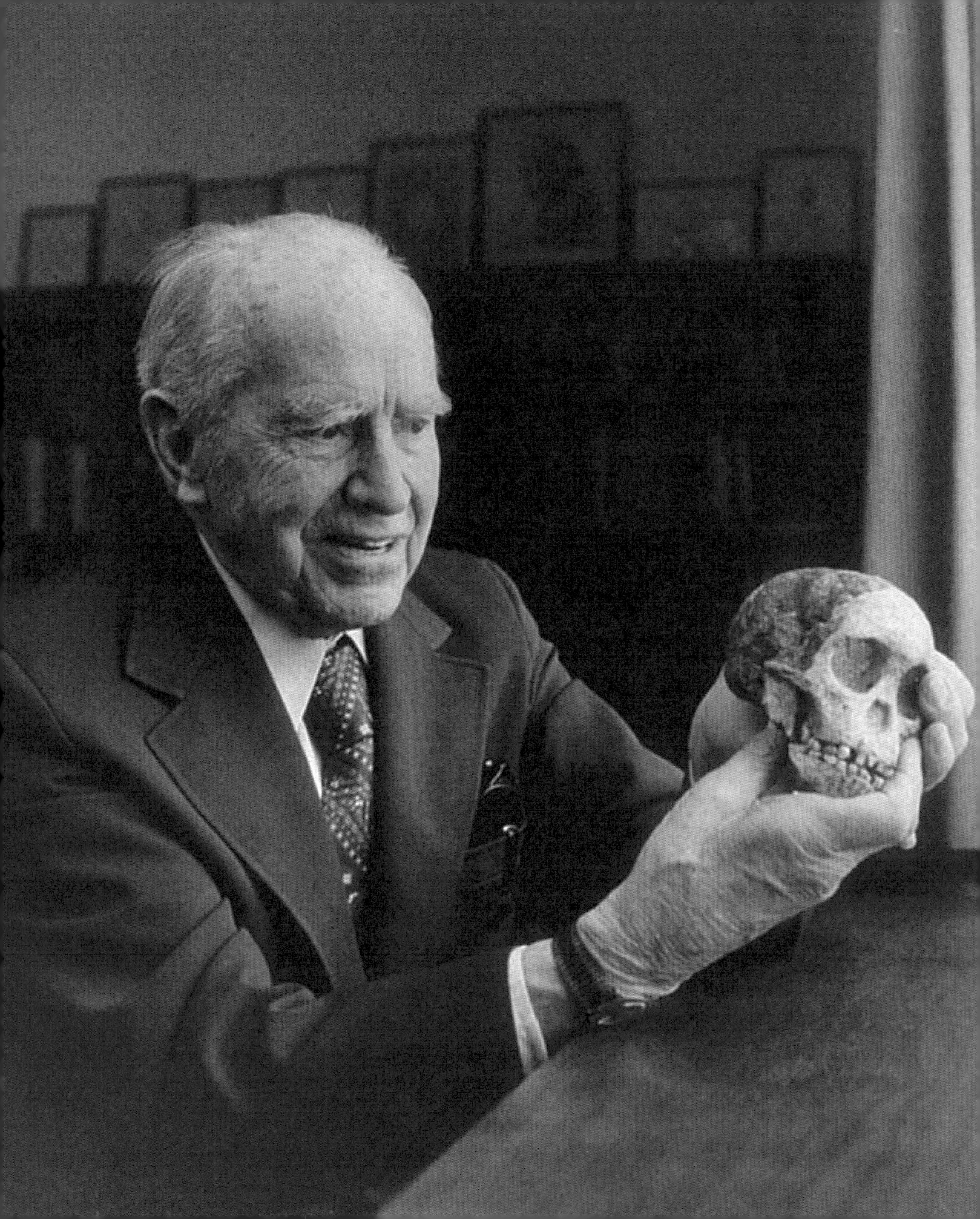

But humans have developed other unique traits, including an egocentric tendency to assume that surviving the torturous and unpredictable evolutionary journey of the last six million years has elevated us to a lofty position above nature; an attitude some anthropologists call 'superorganic'. The idea that we are separate from the power of the natural world is an unrealistic perspective that blinds us to the reality of our vulnerabilities. Incurable diseases, plagues, potential biological disasters, and the whims of an unpredictable planet are poignant reminders that nature continues to play a pivotal role in the survival of all life. At the beginning of the agricultural revolution, humans and domesticated animals constituted 0.1% of the Earth's mammalian biomass. But in just 10,000 years – the blink of a geological eye – that figure has grown to 98%. Our unquenchable hunger for Earth's limited resources has wreaked environmental havoc and causes the extinction of an untold number of species every year.

My African explorations over the last 40 years have not only rewarded me with exceptional discoveries like the 3.2-million-year-old skeleton that came to be known as Lucy, they have also inspired me to reflect on what the past has to say about our species. With more than 500 fossil specimens stretching over nearly 800,000 years now attributed to this species, *Australopithecus afarensis* has become the barometer for evaluating all other hominid specimens. As a young anthropologist, my goal was to find fossils, but I have learned that while the bones are the primary quarry, it is the message they bring us from some long forgotten time that is most meaningful. I have become increasingly intrigued by what Lucy tells us about where we fit into the rhythms of the Earth. Is there something that connects us to nature that transcends time and distance?

Just think – no other species has such a fascination with its origins. No other species has the means to explore and discover the fossilised clues to its beginnings. No other species has so much to learn from its past. But, sadly, no other species has so much to lose by ignoring its genesis.

Despite the predominant, 19th century view that Europe was the finishing school for humanity, Charles Darwin and others pointed to Africa as the cradle of humanity. Raymond Dart's 1924 discovery of the Taung child helped dispel

Raymond Dart and the Taung skull, courtesy Wits University archives.

the Eurocentric view of human origins, and all subsequent hominid fossils have verified Africa as the homeland for humanity. Even the most argumentative kind of *sapiens* – palaeoanthropologists – agree that all the major characteristics constituting humanness premiered in Africa.

Everyone I meet who has been to Africa says they can't wait to go back, that Africa got into their blood. But Africa has always been in our blood, indeed, even in our genes – we now know that our DNA is 99% identical to that of the African chimpanzee. Imagine if we were to receive a message from some far corner of the universe that astronauts had found a hairy, quadrupedal creature so closely related to ourselves? We would spend millions to try to understand what we could learn from this creature about ourselves! So, why do we sit back and do nothing while African ape habitats are being destroyed, and chimps and gorillas become bush meat or souvenirs sold in the streets?

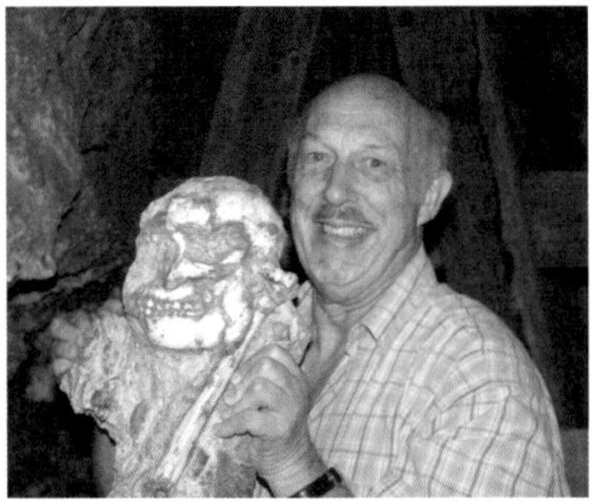

Ron Clarke with 'Little foot', Sterkfontein, 2011, courtesy Ron Clarke and Richard Maire.

I first came to South Africa in the summer of 1970 to study the legendary fossil hominids that I had only read about as a student in America. I recall the exhilaration I experienced when I first saw the Taung child and examined the remarkable treasure trove of hominids at the Transvaal Museum and the University of the Witwatersrand.

Over the years, I have continued to make regular visits to South Africa to study the growing storehouse of fossil hominids, and confer with notables like Dart, Bob Brain, Phillip Tobias, Ron Clarke and others. Nearly every occasion has been overwhelmingly dominated by conversations, discussions and often animated argument about human origins. How many species were there? Which was the true ancestor to later hominids, including modern humans? Which theatre of discovery, eastern or southern Africa was most important and relevant to fleshing out the family tree? When did the genus *Homo* first appear? Were Lucy and the other fossils I was finding in Ethiopia a distinct species from *Australopithecus africanus*? The questions were endless.

RIGHT: Phillip Tobias surrounded by famous original fossil humans such as Cro-Magnon man and Neandertal man in the Musée de l'Homme, Paris. Photograph by Simon Hunt, 1955, courtesy Phillip Tobias.

The 1985 Taung Diamond Jubilee International Symposium, hosted by Wits, was a turning point for me, professionally and personally. I arrived in Johannesburg thoroughly prepared to defend Lucy, *et al.* as a new species, *Australopithecus afarensis*, and to reaffirm her pivotal place on the human family tree. Following

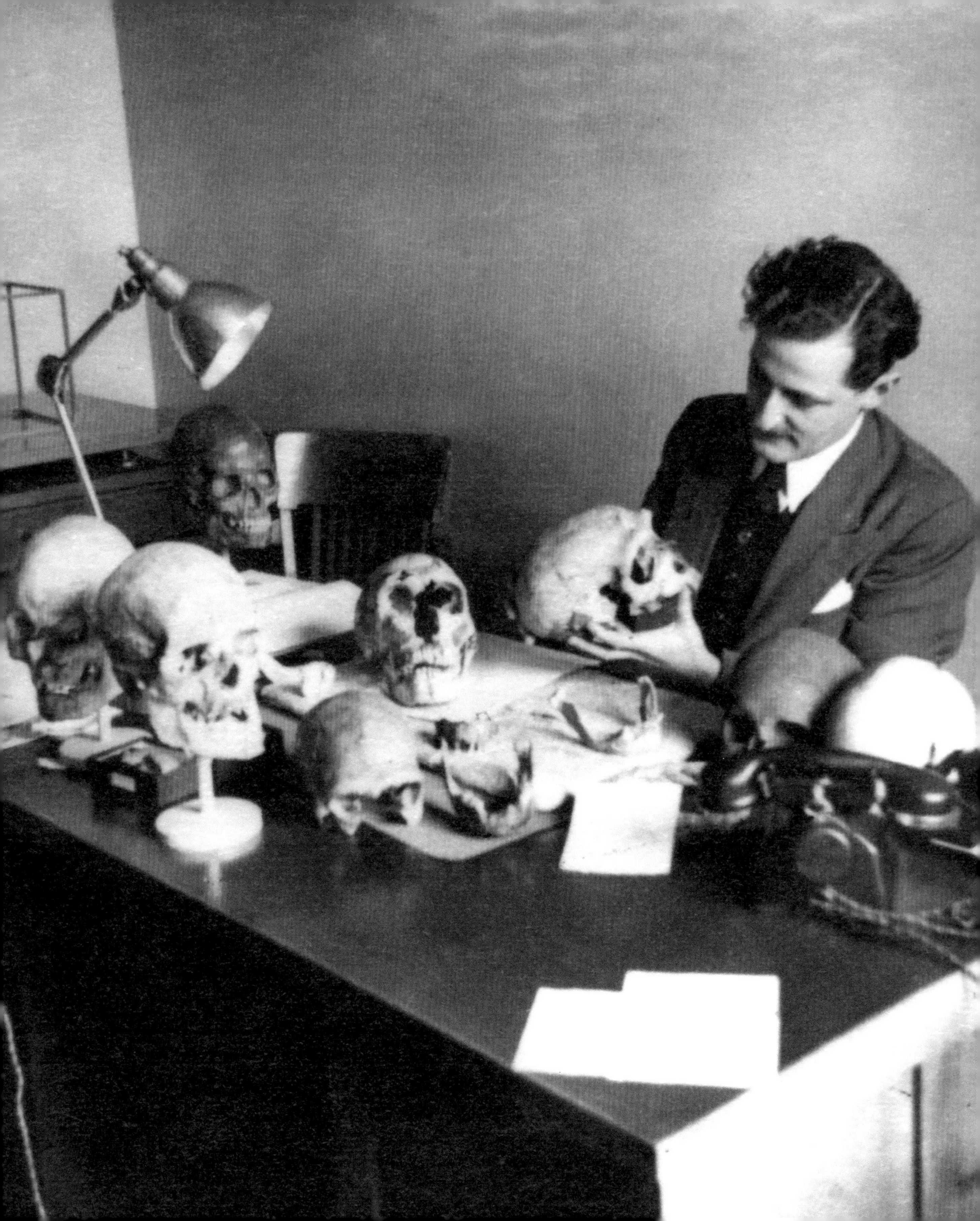

several days of fever-pitch discussion in stuffy lecture halls, we set off on a field excursion to the old Buxton Limeworks at Taung to see the unveiling of a bronze plaque commemorating the initial find in 1924. The bus ride to Bophuthatswana turned out to be surprisingly transformational.

Sometime during the long trip I fell into conversation with a young man, Karel Nel. Now a respected artist and African art specialist, Karel expressed his burning interest in palaeoanthropology and his quest to know our place in nature. After a visit to his family home in Rivonia for tea and an afternoon with him in his vast Wits studio, I knew we would be friends for life. At that time, he was working on a large commission entitled *The Phaedraes*, the gleaming ones, which mapped the energetic field of mind's eye imagery, images initiated by the brain's neural field. Talking to Karel about this work, we forged deep connections because of our shared interest in intelligence and consciousness – those aspects that differentiate us as a species.

Our passion to visit significant remote places in an attempt to understand human, biological and cultural diversity also emerged in these early conversations. We are both 'walk-about men' who see human experience as a continuum, just as I see evolutionary lineages as continuous threads through time. We share an appreciation of the immensity of the universe and the infinity of space, and struggle to understand how and why *Homo sapiens* happened here on Earth.

Bones have meant different things to Karel, the artist, and me, the scientist, but they are important links to understanding our species' past. I look at bones as a principal way of reconstructing the family tree and try to understand why so many branches on that tree went extinct, and only one survived. Karel is interested in extrapolating from the significance placed by our species on burial, and the sacredness often associated with those sites. The bones themselves are often seen as the last link to the deceased, becoming a locus or focal point of beliefs, contact and comfort and a link to the numinous.

Our divergent interests share a reverence for human remains in that they provide clues to our biological and cultural evolution as a species. Karel's interest in sacred and residual sites occasioned visits to Gauguin's grave on the remote

Karel Nel working on *The Phaedras* in his industrial West campus Wits studio, 1985.

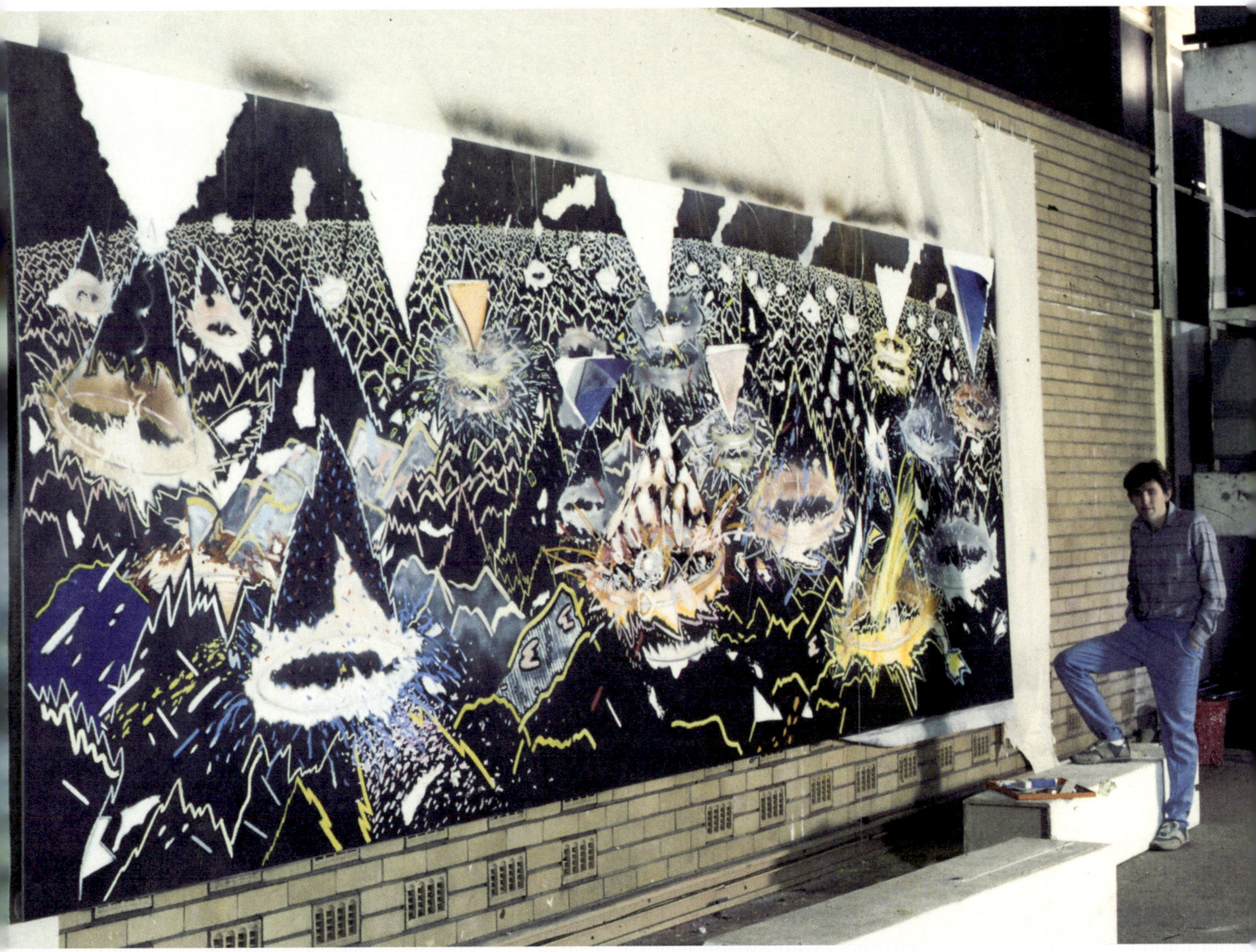

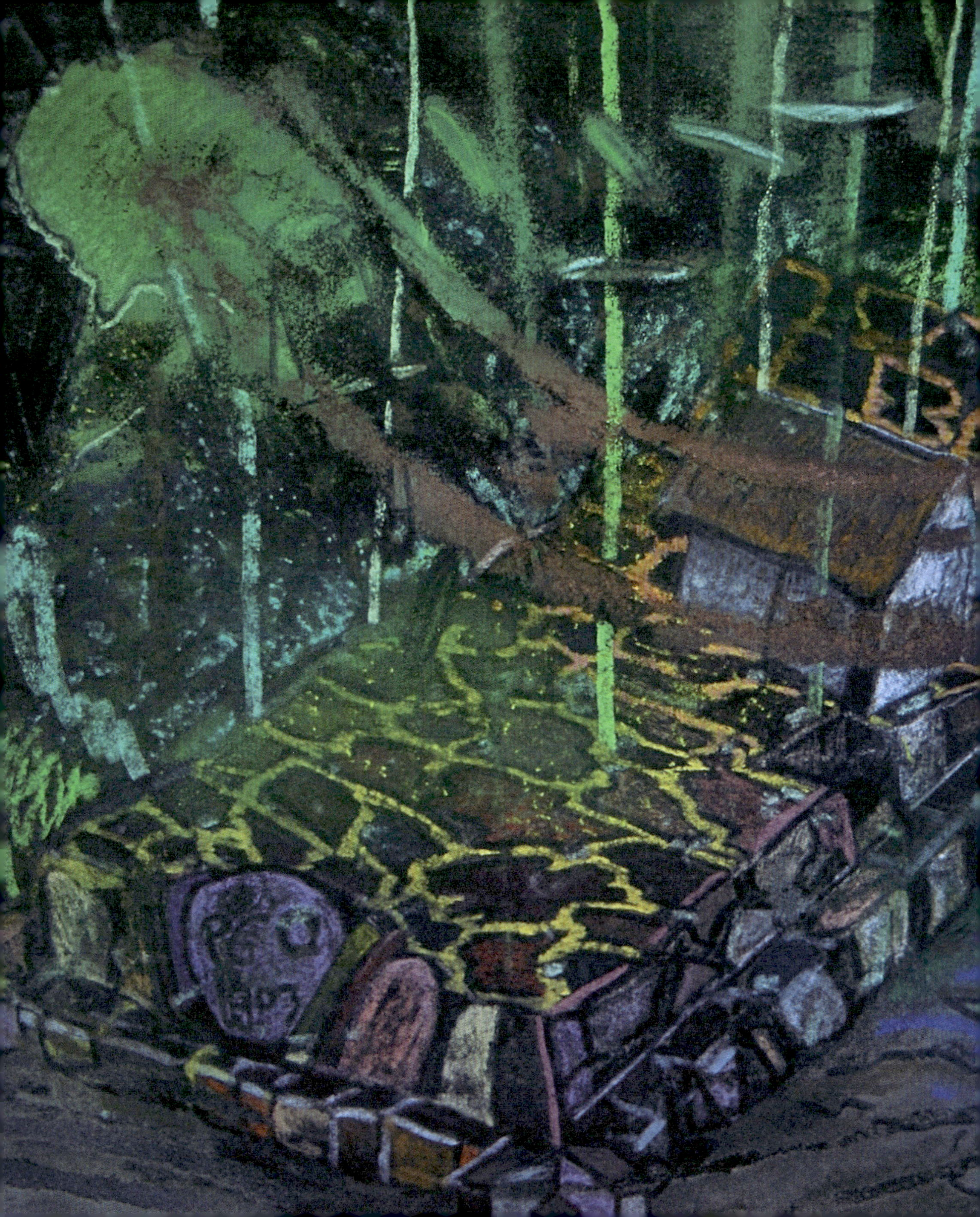

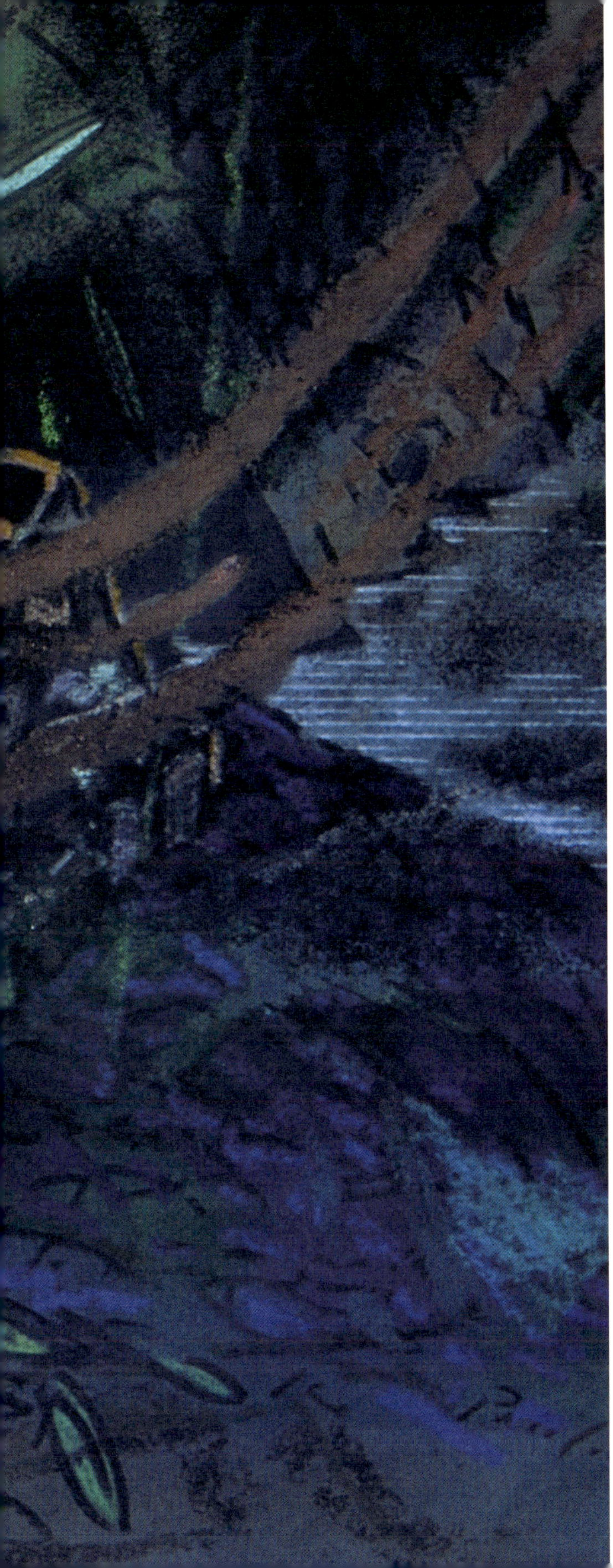

island of Hiva Oa in the Marquesas. His luminous green drawing of Gauguin's resting place on those steep hillside slopes now occupies a large central space in the living room of my San Francisco home.

Karel's overarching interest in the synergy of science and art has consistently been the guiding framework during our common quest to understand the human condition. Where did we come from? is largely an anthropological endeavour, based on an ever-increasing archaeological record. Who are we? is an existential question that reaches beyond the stones and bones. Discoveries now being made on the southern coast of South Africa at Blombos and Mossel Bay are documenting the earliest glimmerings of symbolic behaviour and human innovation. But in our conversations, Karel has challenged me to look at this rudimentary evidence in a broader context and to ponder the innate drive that all humans seem to have to leave a mark of some kind, to record their existence. An aesthetic dimension in our species seems attested to even in the engraved marks in the red ochre found at Blombos, and in the traces of ownership suggested by the rudimentary drilling through shells that would have allowed them to be threaded as adornment or traded. Recent finds of polished pieces of ochre at Mossel Bay are as vital to our understanding of the early human experience as the engineering breakthrough of heat-treating stone to make better tools.

Where are we going? as a species is not simply idle speculation about the cultural and behavioural implications of human capacity, but encompasses wide-ranging evolutionary implications related to issues such as human genetics, ecology, natural resources, custodianship of the

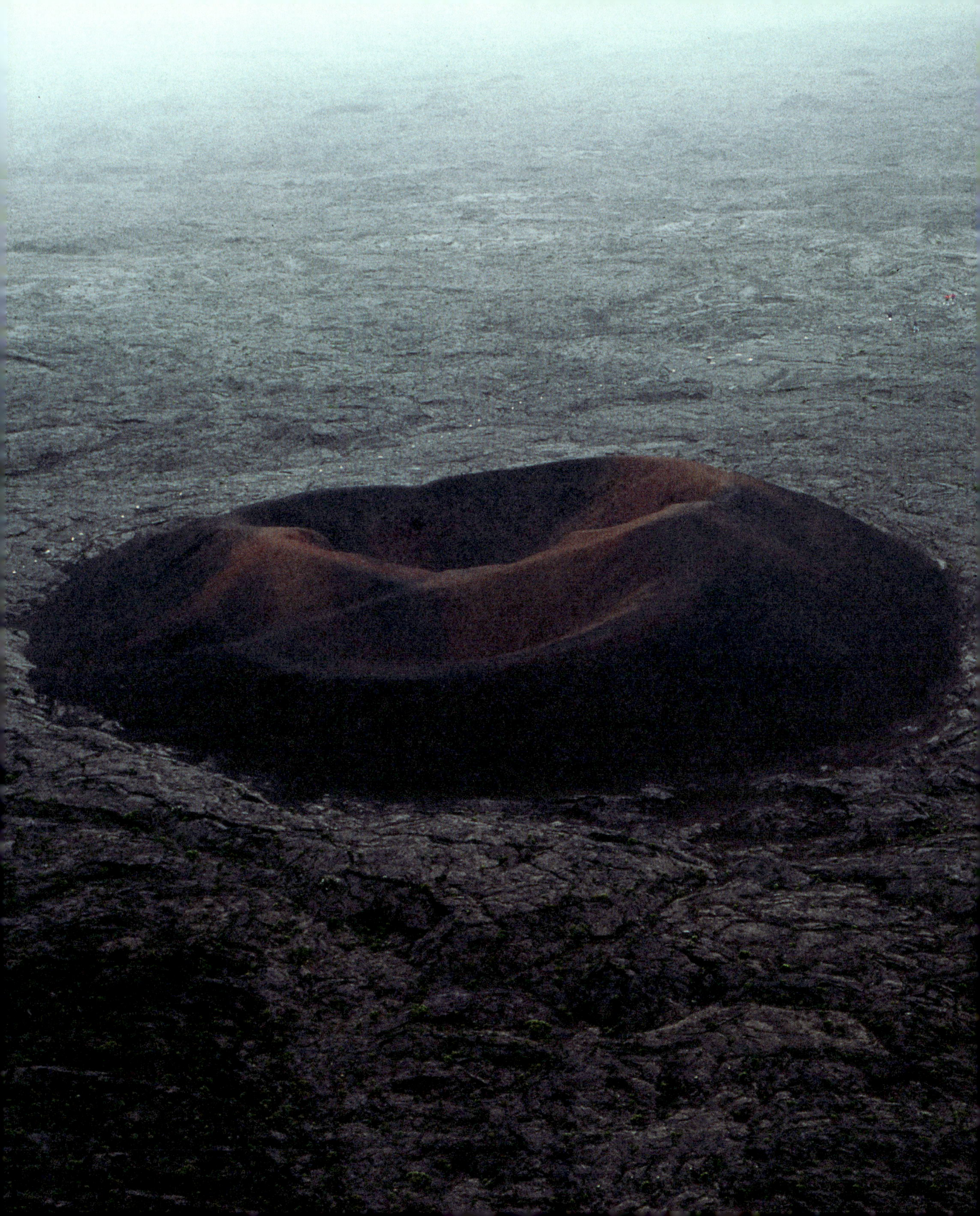

planet, population size, and over-harvesting of the natural world. The existential question includes the extraordinary capacity to trace our way backwards and forwards, and to reflect on both. Early morning tea conversations over the cultural collapse documented on Easter Island and the loss of a knowledge base in Tasmania because of the decimation of the local people, are better mulled over in cross-disciplinary discussions of art, language and archaeology on the consequences of peoples' decisions.

PAGE 110: Karel Nel, *Phosphorescent isle*, pastel and sprayed pigment on bonded fibre fabric, 88 x 220 cm, 1998.

Karel's home in Rivonia, filled with his own art and his collection of sacred art from around the world, is always a rich and stimulating environ for me. He has a painting of a large human skull by the late South African artist, Alexis Preller. The image, in Karel's words, 'glows an uncanny viridian green' and is entitled, *You will never know*. Looking at this evocative piece was a powerful experience when we first saw it in 1985 in the long, low, sleek home of the modernist architect, Tony Doherty, and his wife, Eithné. It remains a constant reminder of our shared interest in the structure of the human skull and the origins of mind and self-reflexive consciousness. Talking about the piece has inspired much speculation about relevance, belonging, purpose and meaning. I have often looked into the empty darkness of fossilised crania and seen nothing, but after late night conversations with Karel, I am prompted to reflect on how those beings engaged with the world millions of years ago. These questions of consciousness relate both to life and death, and are strikingly embodied in the title of the Preller painting, *You will never know*.

Africa, as the crucible of our origins, is always a topic of our discussions from the foggy Berkeley hills, to the pristine beaches of Lamu, the Drakensberg, to Sterkfontein, Kromdraai and Swartkrans. I am reminded of a journey we made years ago to Réunion Island, where we collaborated on a proposed science-art project on Piton de la Fournaise, an active volcano. Here Karel would 're-unite' volcanic rocks from around the globe placing them on the rim of the volcano, reminding us of their single origin in the Earth's molten core. A path through the dormant part of the volcano from the outer to the inner rim was conceived as a timeline that would commence with a cast of a 3.6-million-year-old Laetoli fossil hominid footprint from Tanzania and culminate on the upper edge of the

LEFT: Piton de la Fournaise, the active volcano on Réunion Island. Photograph by Karel Nel, 1996.

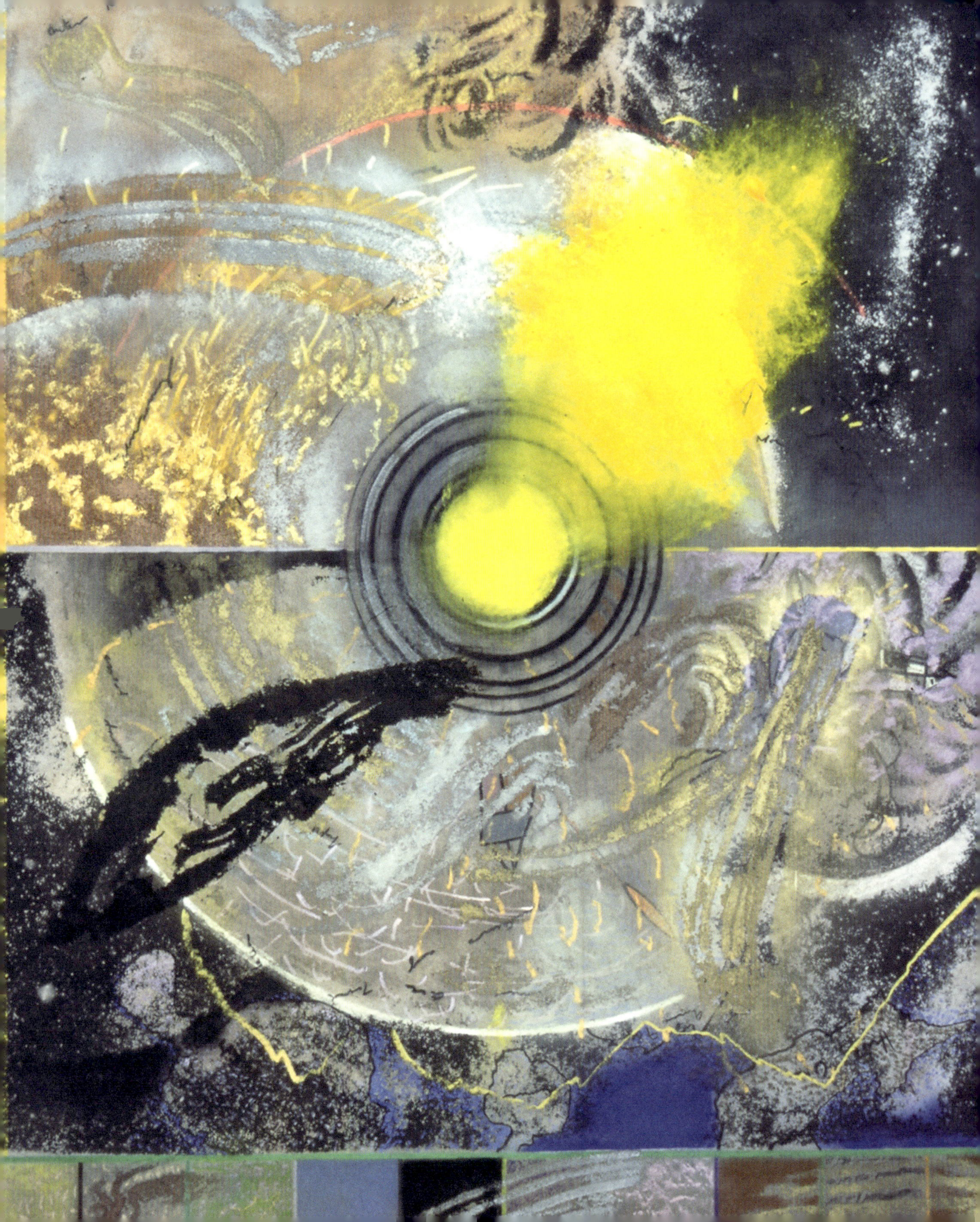

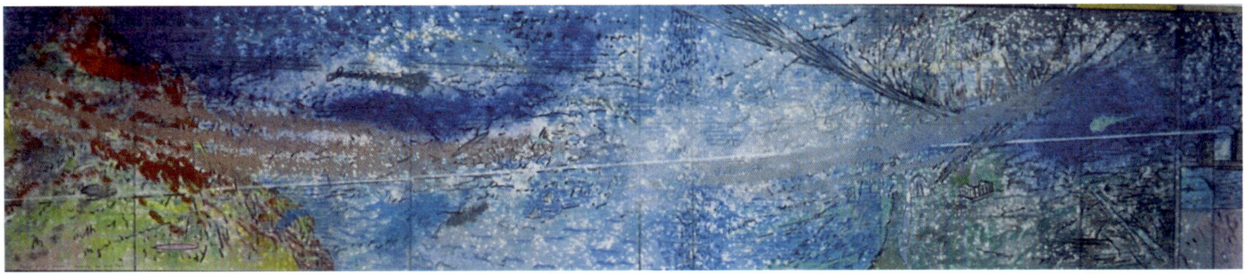

rim with a cast of the astronaut Neil Armstrong's lunar footprint. Along that path, important events in human evolution were to be benchmarked with reminders from 3.6 million years ago to the present.

Our flight to Réunion took us over a bleeding Madagascar where red, lateritic soil was being swept into the Indian Ocean and lemur species become extinct every year from loss of habitat – a result of mining, logging operations and deeply destructive traditional slash-and-burn agriculture. Karel and I have often spoken about the insanity of the human species' irreverent and seemingly unstoppable rape of the natural world.

The poignancy and magic of the natural world emerged during a wonderful hike Karel and I took with friends in the Drakensberg in the early 1990s, not long after Nelson Mandela had completed his long walk to freedom. Our destination was the Ndedema Gorge – one of the richest sites of San rock art in South Africa – and particularly Poacher's Cave, a long shallow overhang where we had secured permission to camp overnight. After enjoying a meal cooked over small fires, and sharing stories of the day's events like our ancestors would have, we crawled into our sleeping bags. Immediately after the last torch was extinguished, the ceiling of the rock overhang lit up with the golden orange of thousands of fireflies that suddenly made a mass exodus to light up the night sky, along with the brilliant stars dotting the black canopy above.

Our conversations have consistently focused on a broad variety of topics ranging from the human capacity for thought, language, art, consciousness and symbolism, to spirituality and transcendence. My appreciation for the fossilised remains of our ancient forbears has expanded far beyond the details of

LEFT: Karel Nel, *Sensory arc and inner isles*, pastel and sprayed pigment on bonded fibre fabric, 240 x 184 cm, 1994.

ABOVE: Karel Nel, *Passing the red isle, Réunion*, pastel and pigment on bonded fibre fabric, 46 x 181 cm, 2000.

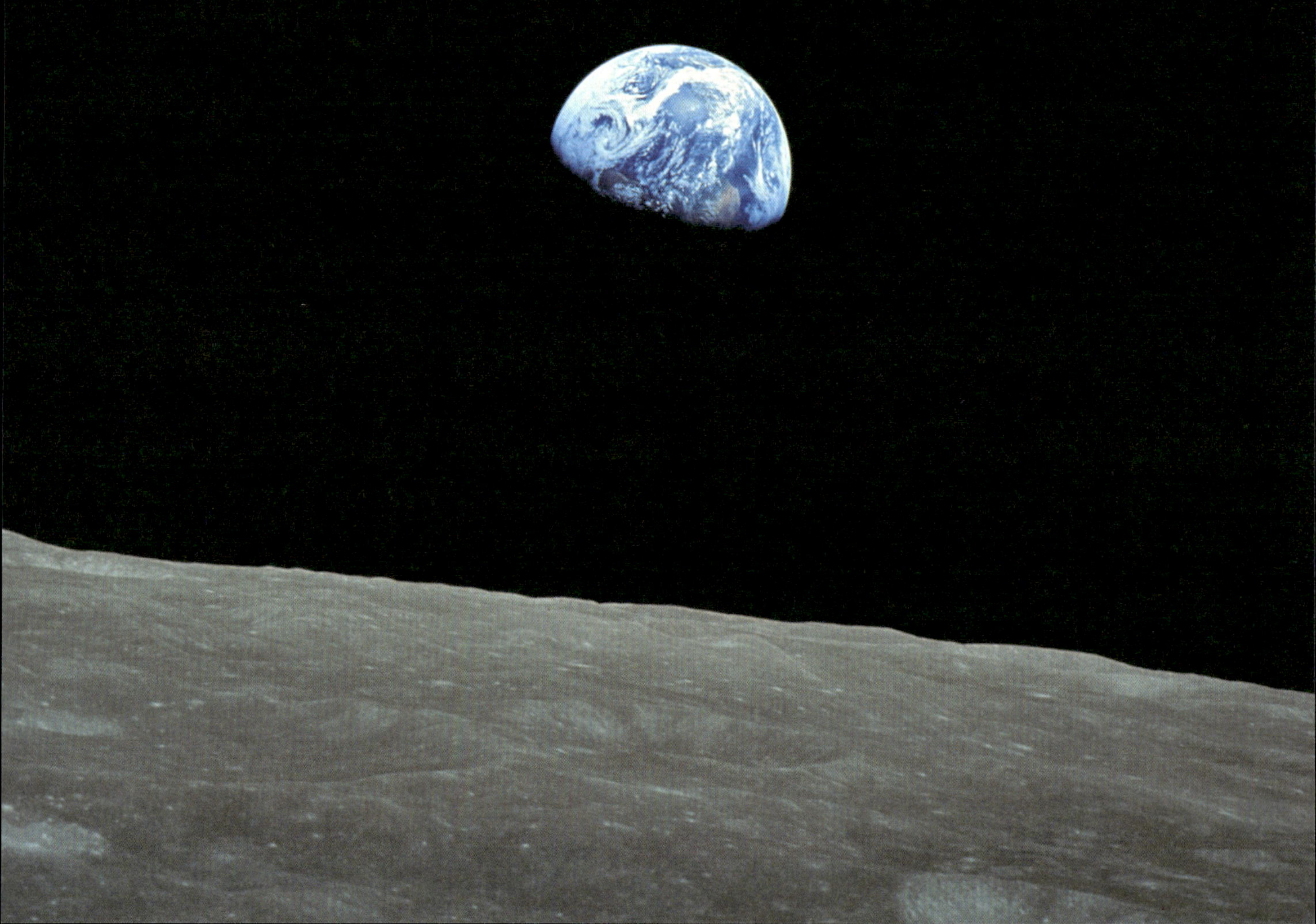

anatomy. With long-dead fossils such introspection has always been a challenge for me, but Karel's gentle nature encouraged me to ponder some of the bigger questions of what it means to be human. The memorable hours of stimulating discussion with him, over more than a quarter of a century, and in a delightful diversity of places, continue to motivate me to think more broadly about the human condition. The fossils are a starting place, but it is imperative that we reflect more intensely about our origins, our place on the planet today and ultimately, our future.

View of the rising Earth that greeted the Apollo 8 astronauts as they came from behind the Moon. Photograph taken by Bill Anders, Apollo 8 crew member, courtesy NASA, 1968.

When I found Lucy in 1974, I did not expect her to become such a powerful ambassador, stimulating people worldwide to reconsider their origins. The Afar tribe who live on the land where Lucy was discovered are devout Muslims, and there is little room in the Koran for the concept of evolution. However, they recognise her significance, and celebrate her as the oldest Afar, the one who gave rise to all humans. In their view, all humans today can be traced back to their tribe. Is this not an example we can learn from?

While we may be the most intelligent animals to walk the Earth, we are not the final resting point of life's three-billion-year adventure; we are still an evolutionary work in progress. In the dawn of this millennium, we must decide how we will treat the planet that has been home for billions of years to every animal, plant, insect and human we have ever studied, patted, swatted or loved. During our brief residence here, we have accomplished great things, but we have also damaged the ozone, destroyed habitats, slaughtered species to extinction and built weapons that could end our noble human legacy. *Homo sapiens*, who learned to measure time, invented the telephone, discovered penicillin and created the most stirring music and paintings, must honour our role as guardians of Earth. Lucy has shown us that we came from the same place. We are one. And only we have the power to influence the outcome of all life on this beautiful, fragile planet.

Notes

1 The title of this essay comes from Paul Gauguin's famous 1897 painting, *D'où Venons Nous/Que Sommes Nous/Où Allons Nous?*

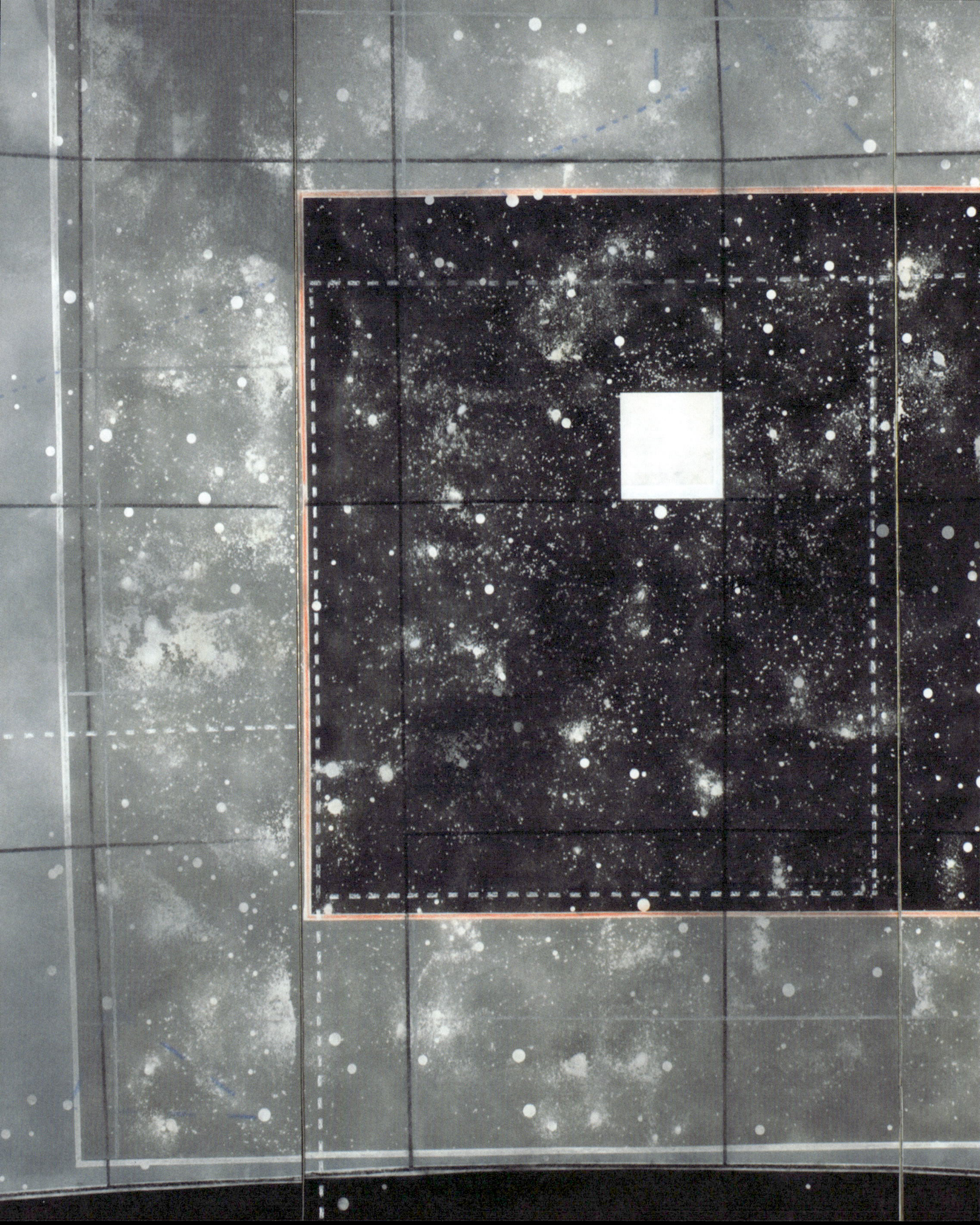

Chapter 7

Matter out of place: four new pieces

Karel Nel

> The choice is still with us, but the civilisation now in jeopardy is all humanity. As the ancient myth-makers knew, we are children equally of the Earth and the sky. In our tenure on this planet we've accumulated dangerous evolutionary baggage – propensities for aggression and ritual, submission to leaders, hostility to outsiders – all of which puts our survival in some doubt. But we've also acquired compassion for others, love for our children and desire to learn from history and experience, and a great soaring passionate intelligence – the clear tools for our continued survival and prosperity. Which aspects of our nature will prevail is uncertain, particularly when our visions and prospects are bound to one small part of the small planet Earth. But up there in the immensity of the Cosmos, an inescapable perspective awaits us.
>
> Carl Sagan, *Cosmos*[1]

Swartkrans/Whitesands

What is one to make of the juxtaposition of the words *Swartkrans* and *Whitesands*? *Swart,* an Afrikaans word, translates as black, and *krans*, as cliff face. Swartkrans, located in the Cradle of Humankind, a world heritage site in South Africa, is the

Karel Nel, *The collapse of time* (detail), sprayed pigment on bonded fibre fabric, 240 x 360 cm, 2008.

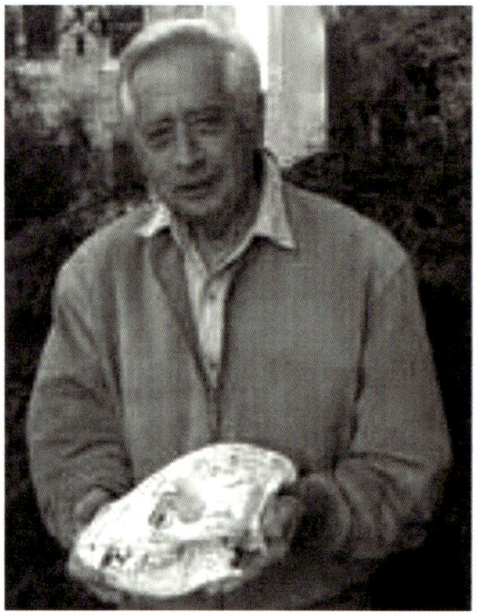

Bob Brain, a pioneer in bringing taphonomic perspectives to human evolutionary studies, 2004, courtesy Bob Brain and the Stone Age Institute.

site of rich reclamation of early hominid fossils and associated bone fragments from animals that were hunted. It is also the site where Bob Brain and his team finally excavated antelope bones that were evidence of the use of fire.

The momentous discovery of these charred remains is recounted by Nicholas Shakespeare in his biography of Bruce Chatwin:

> . . . they had been digging in the west wall for half an hour after lunch when Moenda prised from the earth, alongside an arrangement of three stones, a cracked fragment of antelope bone. Beige white on the outside, blackened on the inside, the bone was speckled with dark patches, as if burned.
>
> George handed it round. It had a soapy feel.
>
> Brain was not a demonstrative man. He had so often set out to find confirmation of his thesis, suffered so many false alarms. But this time, he was visibly moved. 'This bone is remarkably suggestive!'
>
> What they were looking at would eventually be validated, in 1988, as man's first known experimentation with fire. It would predate by 700,000 years the previously oldest find, at Choukoutien in China. 'That was the most convincing evidence for the earliest use of fire, in any human context, anywhere', says Brain. 'It was a very astonishing moment.'[2]

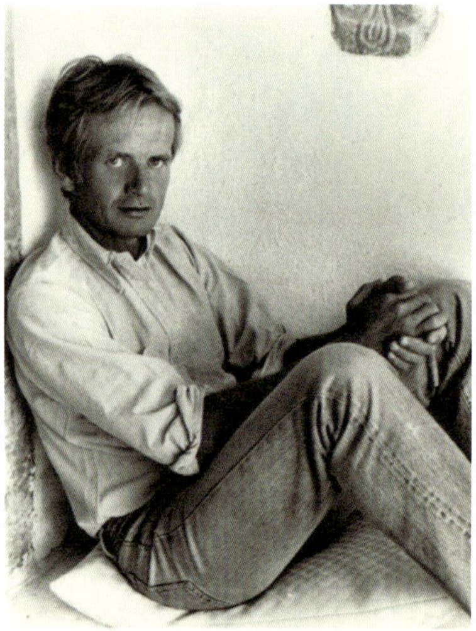

Portrait of Bruce Chatwin. Photograph by Jane Bown, courtesy Jane Bown/Guardian News & Media Ltd, 1987.

Chatwin himself had recorded his own account of that day:

> When visiting the excavation at Swartkrans with Bob Brain, one of the questions uppermost in my mind was man's use of fire: the myth of Prometheus is absolutely crucial, to my mind, in understanding the condition of the First Man – since it was with fire that Man could adequately protect himself at night from the predators.[3]

The primordial ability to control the energy of fire and its relationship to protection is played out differently in the 20th century at Whitesands in New Mexico. Here the 'controlled' atomic testing unleashed unimaginable energy and light with enormous destructive potential – energy later to be directed at Hiroshima

Swartkrans landscape. Photograph by Boyce Rensberger, 1973.

Karel Nel, *Swartkrans/Whitesands*, site-specific dusts, 60 x 150 cm each, 2011

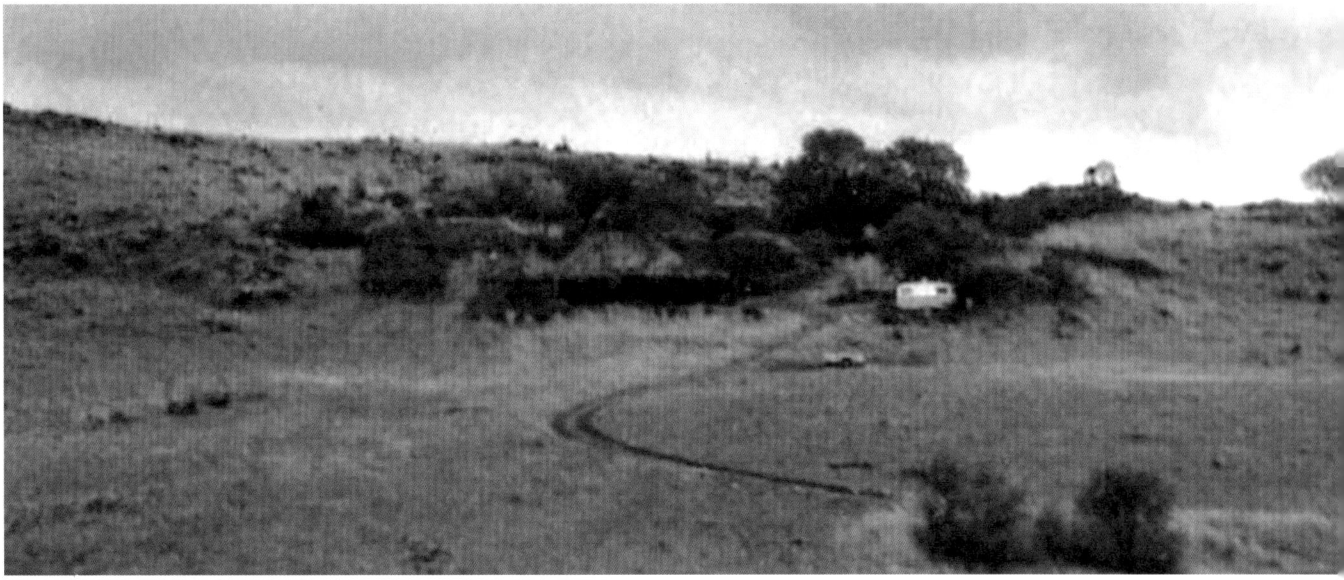

SWART KRANS

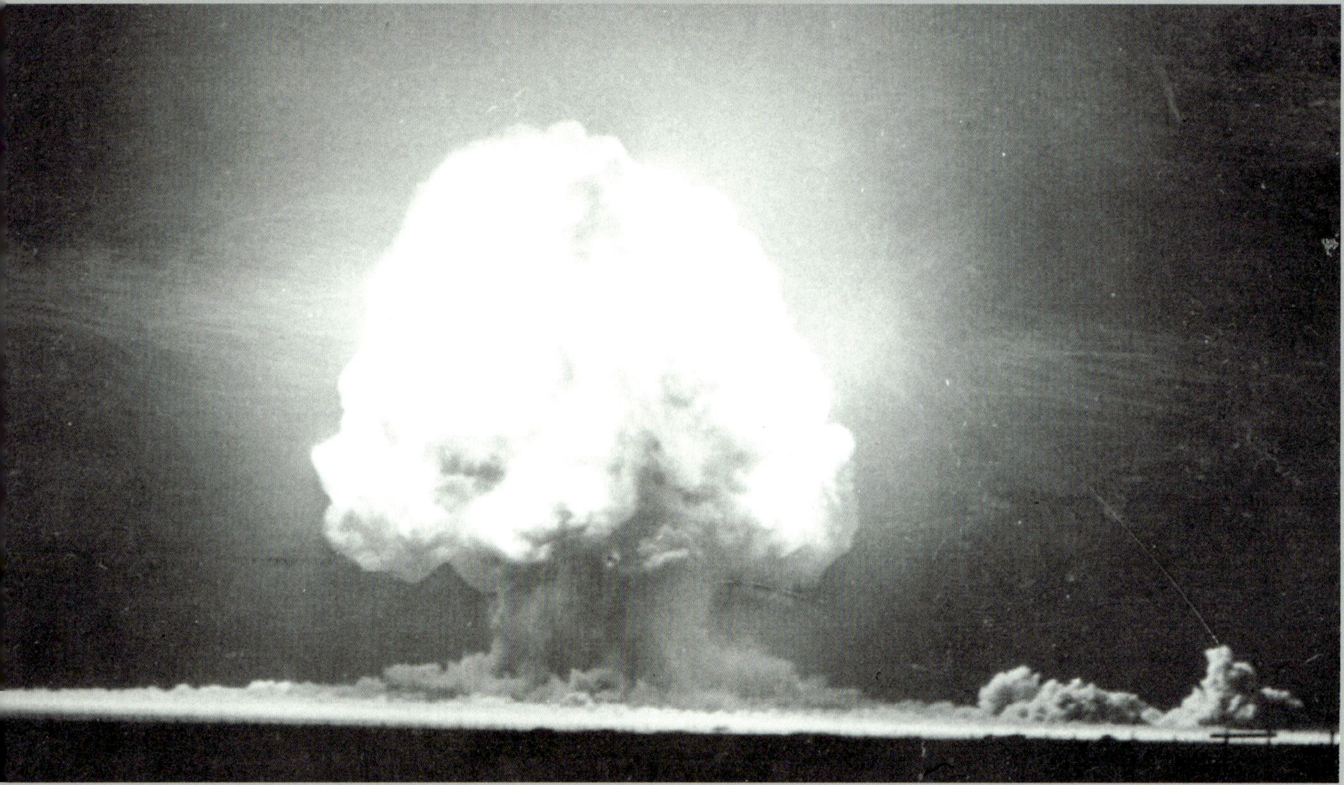

WHITE SANDS

and Nagasaki: our species ironically 'protecting' itself from its predator self, with disastrous consequences.

Whitesands, Trinity test, New Mexico, July 16, 1945, courtesy of the National Nuclear Security Administration, Nevada Site Office.

In contrast to the blackened bones of Swartkrans, at Whitesands, the heat trace left from the atomic blast is a vitrified glass-like surface on the ground.

These two fire traces are searing cause for speculation on the advancement of our species since harnessing the use of fire in the caves of Swartkrans.

Perhaps it was not only with fire that early hominids protected themselves. Chatwin suggested that 'it was through language that the earliest hominids saved themselves', and the evidence of fire has suggested to Brain the 'perfectly valid speculation' that language, and so storytelling, might have evolved from a need to issue warnings about our predators. 'Language came into being,' Brain says, 'out of a need for far more precise communication and identification of objects and circumstances, and for more elaborate audible signals.'[4]

In this contemporary moment, the visual and material juxtaposition of the words 'Swartkrans' and 'Whitesands' embodies a profound warning or caution. Far more than evoking specific sites, the fields of dust together with the engraved words prompt the mind to reflect on the creative and destructive impulses and behaviour of our species, enabling us to reflect on the long evolutionary track that we have travelled between then and now.

All work, artistic and scientific, is to some extent driven by personal impulses. Most of my work is autobiographical. Many of my dust works, as in *Cultural Ground*, map my yearly travels between South Africa, London, New York and other more remote destinations. They are in some senses a diary and a meditation as well as a new form of landscape painting.

Sterkfontein/Rietfontein

I live on Rietfontein Road in Rivonia, the suburb that became famous – or infamous – because of the Rivonia trial, which put Nelson Mandela and the core of the ANC into prison on Robben Island for almost three decades. It is a 40-minute drive to Sterkfontein, Kromdraai and Swartkrans. These names – Rietfontein and

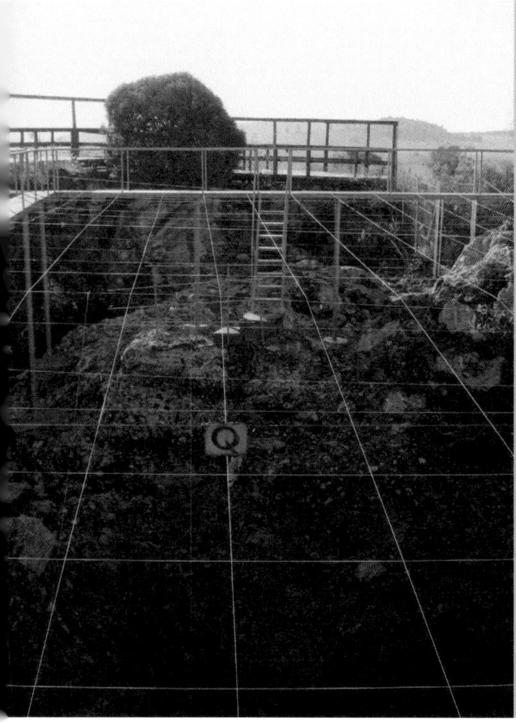

LEFT: Sterkfontein excavation site in the Cradle of Humankind. Photograph by Sally Gaule, 2006.

CENTRE: Karel Nel, *Sterkfontein/Rietfontein*, site specific dusts, 150 x 150 cm each, 2011

RIGHT: Karel Nel working in his Rietfontein road studio, Rivonia, Johannesburg. Photograph by John Hodgkiss, 2011.

Sterkfontein – have inhabited my imagination since I was a boy and continue today to evoke a powerful sense of home and place. How else could it be, when palaeoanthropology and genetics pinpoint the very origins of our species to just around the corner?

Rietfontein Road is where I built my studio, and it's the place of my upbringing. It is here that the formation of my broad interests in art, anthropology and the palaeosciences took root. Here is where, as a 16-year-old, I read *The Phenomenon of Man*, Teilhard de Chardin's sophisticated synthesis of the relationship between geology, palaeoanthropology and spirituality: the book reflects his insights into the complexification of consciousness and its relationship to evolution, and in some way too, reflects his own complex mental biography. I was intrigued that Chardin, who died in 1955, the year of my birth, had visited Sterkfontein in 1951: each somehow brought to the same place, at different times, both exploring the evolution of consciousness and just missing the chance to speak! Rietfontein

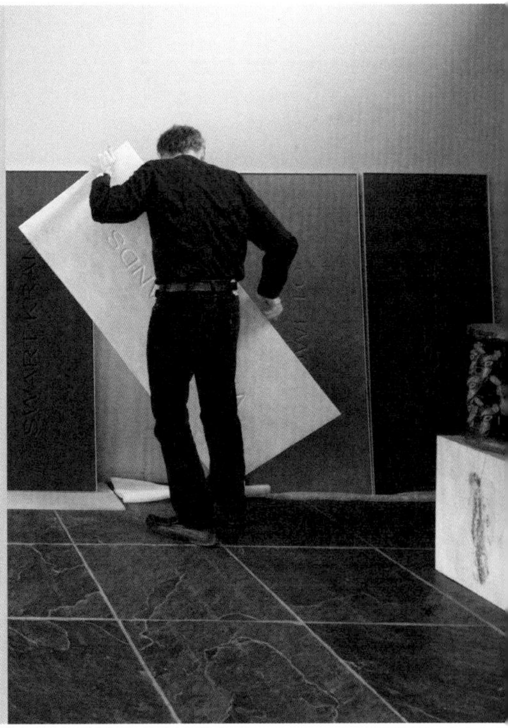

Road is also the place where I came to know, over the years, several scholars and scientists who were drawn to this region of Africa, and specifically the Cradle of Humankind, and with whom I have been fortunate to have walked and talked at these significant sites. The privilege of knowing Phillip Tobias, Ron Clarke and Donald Johanson, along with many other palaeoanthropologists who have worked and visited in this region, would not have been possible had I lived, say, in the Cape. Place makes us who and how we are, and *Sterkfontein/Rietfontein* is a tribute to that idea.

Sterkfontein/Rietfontein is my attempt to understand my own place in the continuum of deep time. It contains the questions we might ask about our relationship with our species, and with how we, as modern humans, connect to and reflect on our place within this immense trajectory of time. For me, it is a deeply reflective work, absent of image, and like a diary, annotates the personal and evolutionary journey from Sterkfontein to Rietfontein, both cool places, places of mud.

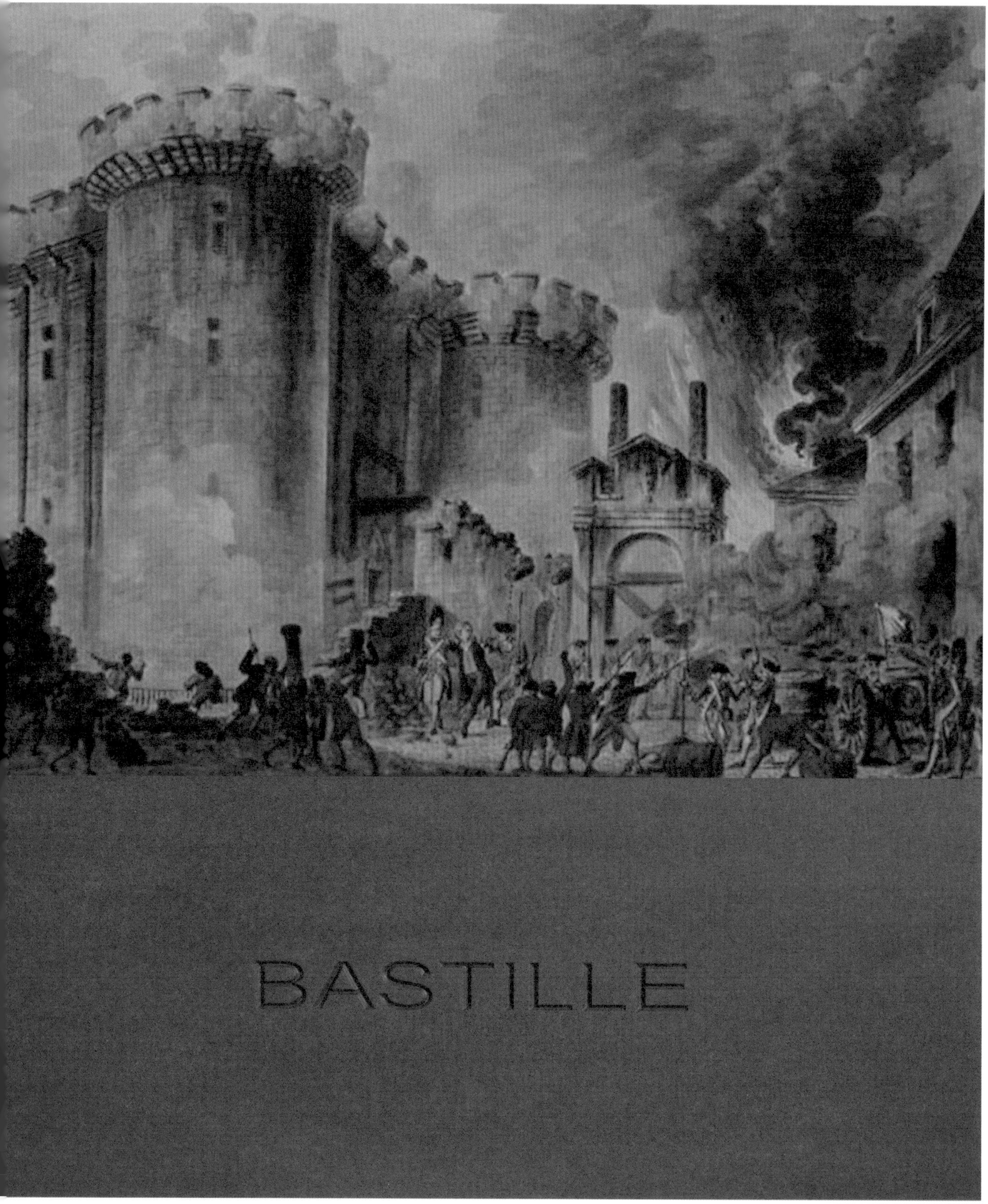

BASTILLE

Bastille/Soweto

TOP: Jean-Pierre Houël, *Storming of the Bastille*, watercolour, 37.8 x 50.5 cm, 1789, courtesy Bibliothèque Nationale de France.

BOTTOM: Karel Nel, *Bastille/Soweto*, site-specific dusts, 60 x 150 cm each, 2011.

> Those who cannot remember the past are condemned to repeat it.
>
> George Santayana, *The Life of Reason, Volume 1, 1905*

Bastille/Soweto is a rumination on the nature of our species, not based on the fossil record this time, but on the iterated patterns of our solutions to social interactions, and the repeated power strategies used to control them. Strategies that have helped develop our sense of community at times have, at others, acted as unbearable constraints leading to violent disruption.

The birth of democracy, the evolution of an egalitarian society and the creation of a constitution that protects human rights – to move from inequality and an imbalance of resources to a civil society in which all have a voice and a right to be: these are the cherished norms to which many societies strive.

The Bastille was, as most of us know, a medieval fortress and infamous prison in Paris. Its destruction, which served as the flashpoint of the French Revolution, created its iconic status in France, and in world imagination today. The Bastille was a symbol of untenable oppression during the reign of Louis XVI and Marie Antoinette. A massive disproportionate imbalance of wealth and power between the aristocracy and peasant class galvanised the masses in a revolt that is today legendary. Initially disordered but growing to a critical mass, the unrest spilled over with a momentum that was unstoppable. It swept away the old order, deeply questioned the dynamics around power and economics, and challenged that society and its power to the core.

The storming of the Bastille was a blazing marker on the road to democracy. So hated and threatening was its physical presence that it was razed to the ground by the revolutionary masses.

Closer to home and to the present, the impact of critical mass action is powerfully captured in Peter Gabriel's lyrics, the tribute he wrote in memory of Steve Biko, the political activist tortured and killed in South African police custody in 1977, just one year after the 1976 social uprising that began in Soweto.

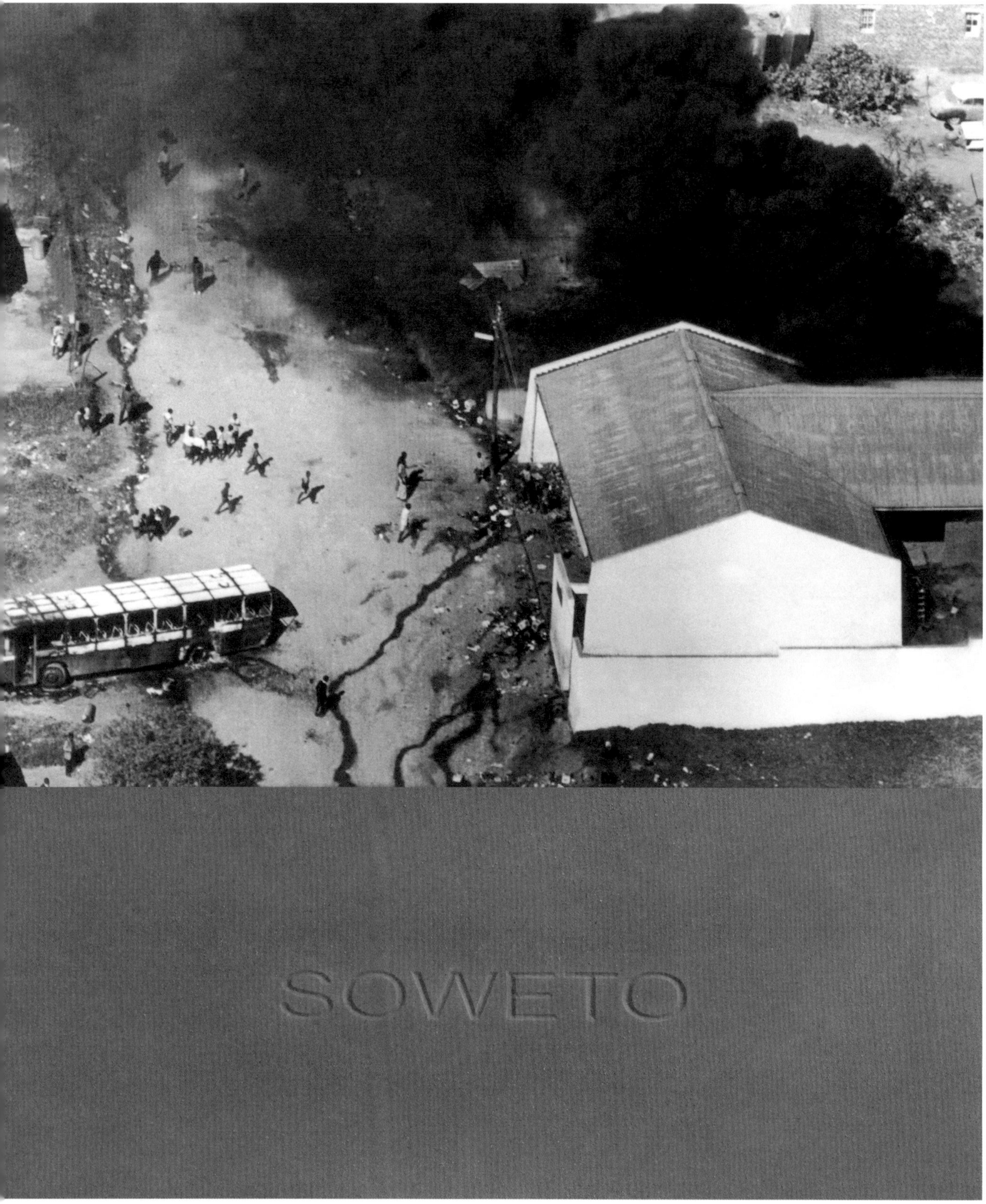

SOWETO

You can blow out a candle,
But you can't blow out a fire
Once the flames begin to catch
The wind will blow it higher.

Peter Gabriel, *Biko*

TOP: Soweto riots, burning warehouse, photograph, 1976, courtesy Keystone-France/Gamma-Keystone/Getty images.

BOTTOM: Karel Nel, *Bastille/Soweto*, site-specific dusts, 60 x 150 cm each, 2011.

In the late 1950s and early 1960s, Mandela and central members of the ANC had called for the end of colonialism, apartheid and white domination, only to be accused of high treason during the Rivonia Trial and thrown into prison, silenced and isolated. Mandela's statement during the trial reflects this tragic irony:

> During my lifetime, I have dedicated myself to this struggle of the African people. I have fought against white domination, and I have fought against black domination. I have cherished the ideal of a democratic and free society in which all persons live together in harmony and with equal opportunities. It is an ideal which I hope to live for and to achieve. But if needs be, it is an ideal for which I am prepared to die.[5]

That he should have been incarcerated for ideals such as these is almost beyond conception just half a century later, but this history reflects the fear of change and of loss of power and status of whites, the dominant class at the time. The dramatic disparity in wealth and power in South Africa, created by a punitive racism, had been further exacerbated by being written into apartheid laws that governed people's lives, jobs, movements and ownership of property.

The struggle to transform and subsequently to overthrow the Nationalist government and its restrictive laws was long, tragic and courageous. It took time for the critical mass to build up, and it was ultimately a language issue around compulsory tuition in Afrikaans that finally ignited the youth of Soweto to tip the balance of power, making the country ungovernable.

As with the revolutionary French example, the sweeping away of an oppressive system and the development of a new social order is often explosive, disruptive and may take many years to find its true bearings. Mandela's release,

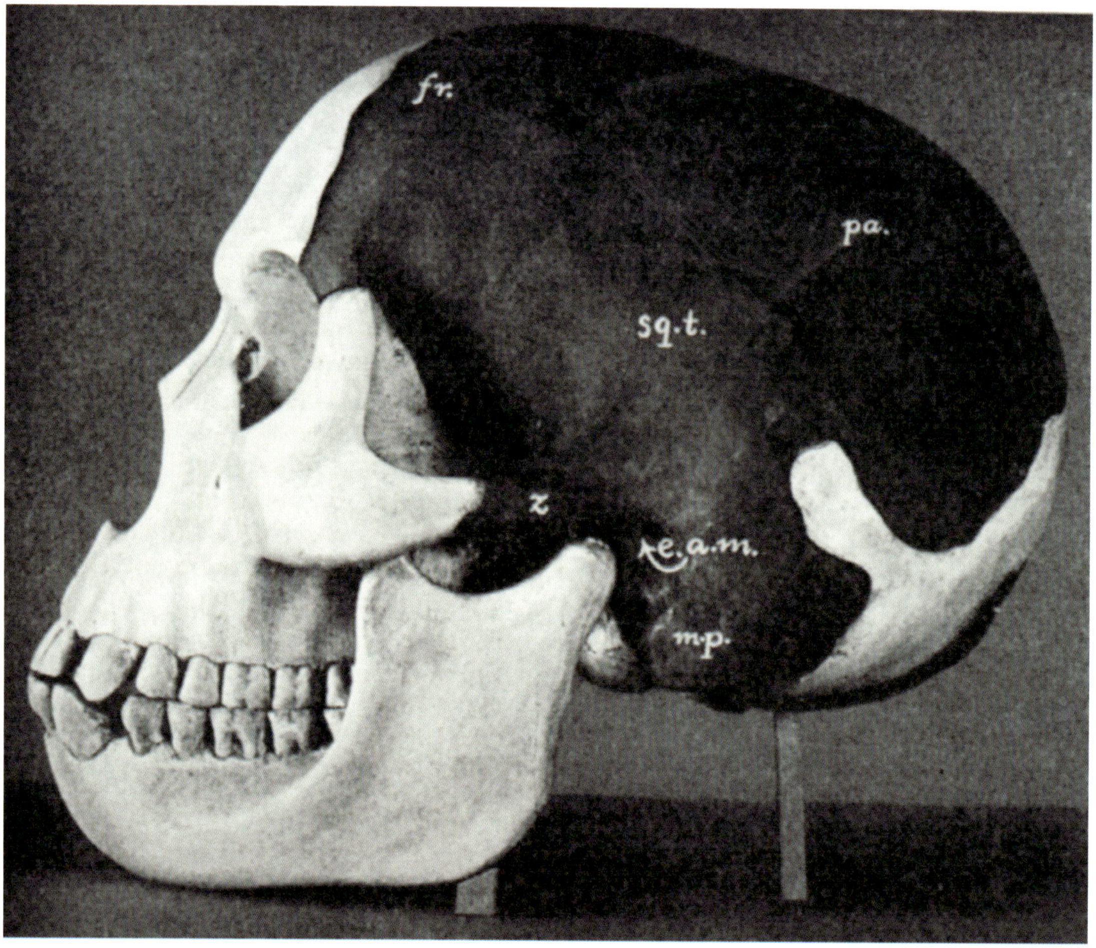
fr.
pa.
sq.t.
z
e.a.m.
m.p.

PILTDOWN

the release of all political prisoners, the unbanning of political parties, the first free and fair election and the new Constitution followed. But the site of the pupils' confrontation with the police marked Soweto permanently and consolidated that moment in the public imagination as the catalyst of change.

'Let the dust settle' is a phrase that signals a disturbance, but it also suggests that the disturbance needs time to be processed. Literally, in the past, if you visited Soweto at dusk, the air was a soft golden hue, the result of dense urbanisation, dusty roads and gardens of sand. Metaphorically, the pupils of Soweto, with their actions, drew a line in the sand, and the dust of those tumultuous events is still in the process of settling.

These two words 'Bastille' and 'Soweto' resound with the creative and destructive forces that lead to change and transformation.

TOP: Model of the skull of Piltdown Man, as reconstructed by Arthur Smith Woodward, 1914, courtesy Photos.com/Getty images.

BOTTOM: Karel Nel, *Taung/Piltdown*, site-specific dust/Fuller's earth (fake theatrical dust), 35 x 150 cm each, 2011

Taung/Piltdown

Taung and Piltdown signal a different power struggle. The presence of the Taung fossil now undeniably locates the origins of humankind in southern Africa. But the Piltdown fossil 'discovery' for many years was seen as the keystone specimen in the model that placed hominid development firmly within Europe, and particularly in England. Despite its questionable idiosyncrasies, the fossil was nonetheless given much credence among the scientific community, indicating how neatly it fitted Eurocentric presuppositions about human evolution at the time. As humans, we are indeed so mesmerised by our own suppositions and projections that at times we are unable to see an alternative view. Although the Piltdown man eventually turned out to be a palaeoarchaeological hoax, its history is a fascinating example of the struggle between that which one does – and doesn't – want to know.

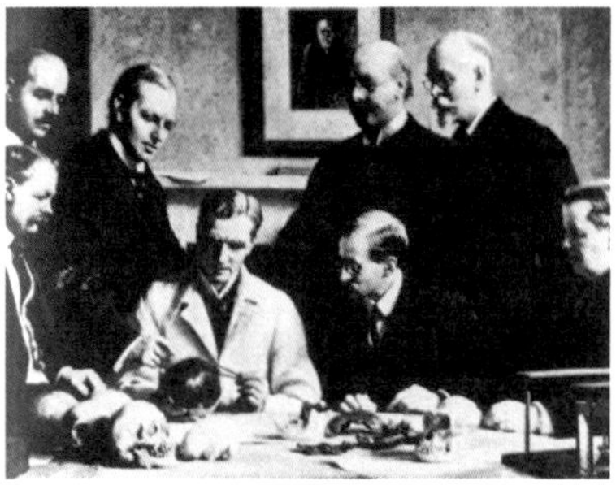

Photograph of John Cooke's, *The Piltdown committee,*
(Back row from left): F.O. Barlow, G. Elliot Smith, Charles Dawson, Arthur Smith Woodward
(Front row): A.S. Underwood, Arthur Keith, W.P. Pycraft, and Sir Ray Lankester, 1915, courtesy of Royal Geological Society archives.

Raymond Dart's discovery and description of the Taung child was to radically challenge the significance of the Piltdown specimen. Its announcement was thus understandably greeted with hostility and then largely ignored for several decades.

The breccia dust collected from the Buxton Limeworks at Taung is laid down

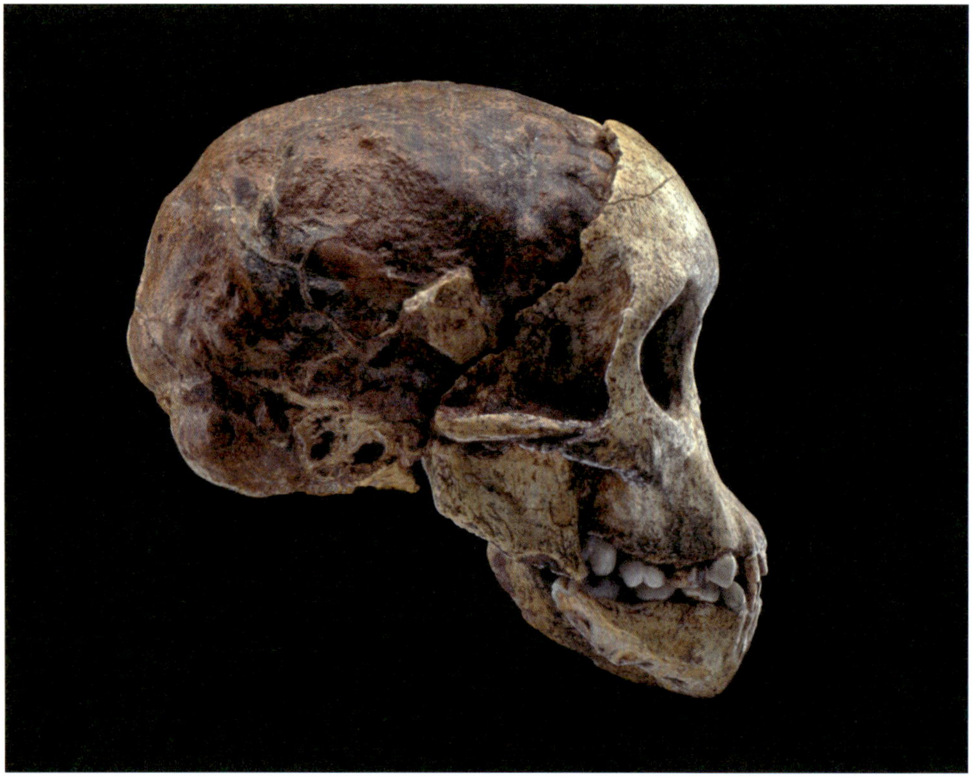

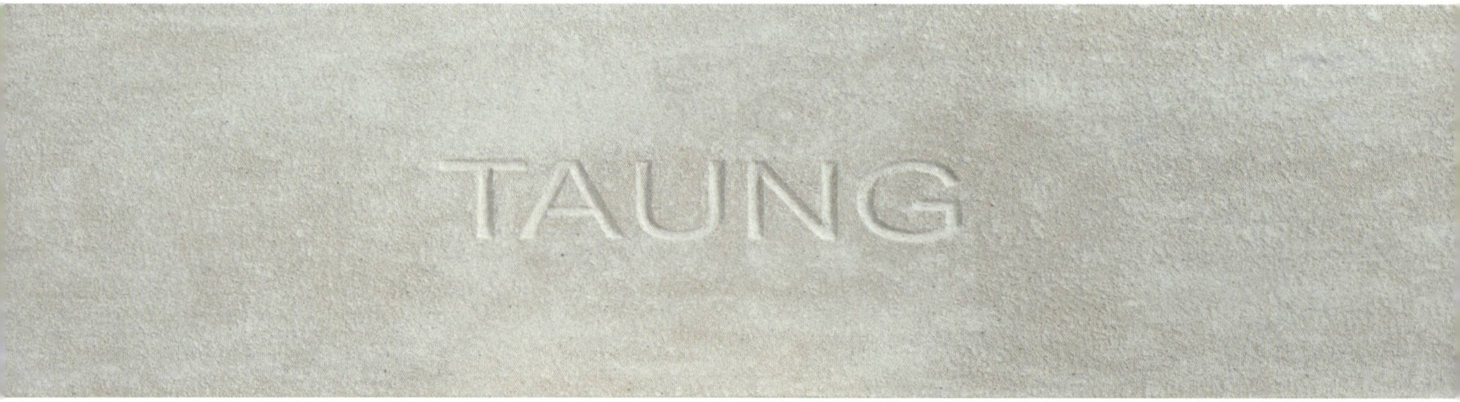
TAUNG

side by side with theatrical dust, a product made specifically for illusion on stage. It is literally fake dust.

The two panels of dust in *Taung/Piltdown* distil an enormous global power struggle – between the 'centre' and 'periphery' of knowledge, between the 'civilised' and the 'primitive' – in laying claim to our topographical origins.

It is always easier to consider two things than one, to compare and contrast, and to find the intersections and insights that comparative looking and thinking yield. These four new works embody this strategy: each one represents a pair of ideas, and displacements, which direct our attention to significant moments and insights into human behaviour and impulses, across time and place. Each of these works, which edit out almost every aspect of the visual to focus on the mental, the conceptual, nevertheless functions as a contemporary memento mori. The works serve as memorials, comprising the dust of places made significant by the death of one or many.

The displacement between two ideas, or two places, or matter out of place alerts the eye/mind to act on knowledge and thought to create meaning in the material world. That these four works function in this way renders them simultaneously explicit and implicit. They are images of absence and presence. The plain dusty panels prompt a complex tracery of mental impressions and associations, unleashing an unbounded response, liberating the mind to create a series of connections in a non-linear matrix. The works challenge the idea of the work of art as a window to the world, allowing the viewer to enter only mentally. This abstract process of viewing enables us to excavate the pertinent relationships between one idea and another, one place and another, one time and another. In this sense, each work also functions as a *momento morum*, a reminder of the impact that our human actions – considered and ill-considered – have upon ourselves and the planet.

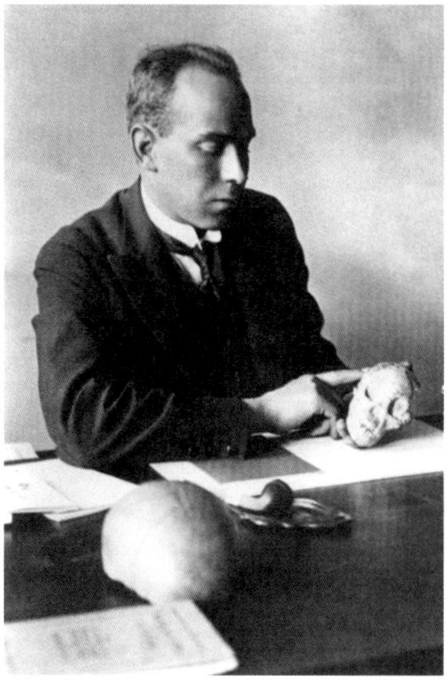

Raymond Dart, 1925. Photograph courtesy Barlow Rand and Phillip Tobias.

Notes

1 *Cosmos: Carl Sagan*. 2002. DVD. Cosmos Studios. Produced by Richard Wells.

2 Shakespeare, N. 1999. *Bruce Chatwin*. London: Harvill Press in association with Jonathan Cape. p. 3.

3 ibid.

4 ibid. p. 5.

5 Mandela, N.R. 1995. *Long Walk to Freedom: The Autobiography of Nelson Mandela*. Boston, New York, London: Back Bay Books. p. 368.

LEFT TOP: *A. africanus*, Taung, Sterkfontein, skull, lateral right. Photograph by David Brill, 1985, courtesy Medical School, University of the Witwatersrand.

LEFT BOTTOM: Karel Nel, *Taung/Piltdown*, site-specific dust/Fuller's earth (fake theatrical dust), 35 x 150 cm each, 2011

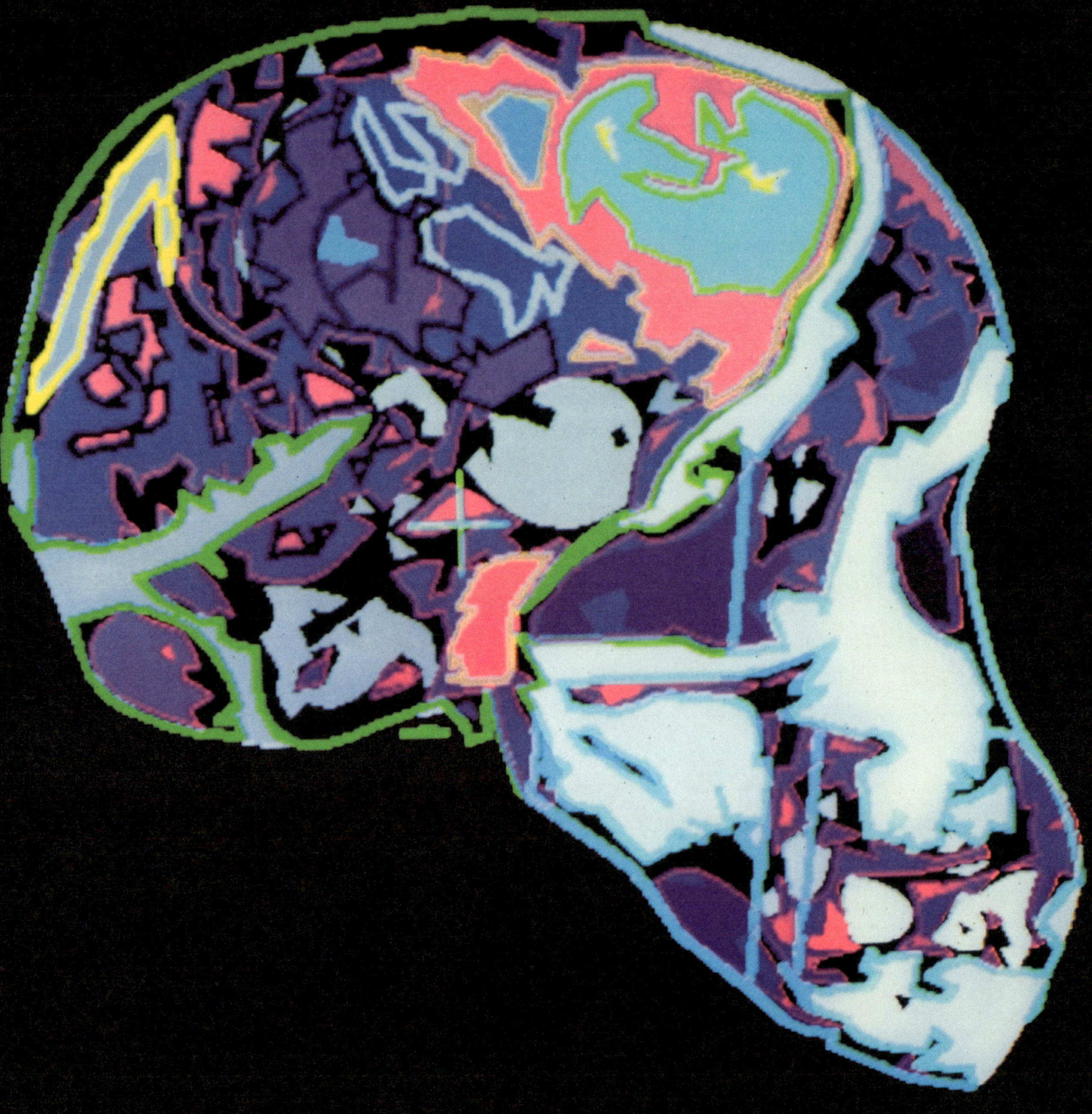

Chapter 8

Cartographer of consciousness: Karel Nel

Elizabeth Burroughs

Both curtains were sucked out of the high window. Karel clambered up onto the bed to see what had caused their sudden exit. The curtains blew back in as he peered out. The dust from the vegetable beds was jumping up into the air. At the mighty explosions, I sprang up to look out too. The ruddy dust was rising in the early morning light. As the sand gradually settled, we too settled back into the routine of breakfast and preparation for school. The 7 o'clock news on Grandpa's radio announced that a series of massive blasts had rocked the AE&CI dynamite factory at Modderfontein a little earlier, breaking windows in the surrounding areas. The hectic clamour and then the softly sifting reddish dust had signalled, whether real or imagined, insurrection – tectonic shifts in our lived reality.

Only relatively recently did Karel and I speak about the impact of growing up in Rivonia in the early 1960s, in the time before it hit the headlines. The sensational arrests and subsequent trial that made our village infamous, formed the ambiguous culmination of anxieties which had pervaded our household in the year or so before Nelson Mandela, Walter Sisulu, Govan Mbeki and their comrades were captured in the police raid on Liliesleaf Farm. When we talked about the impact of those early experiences, I said I had lost any sense of future, and with it, any sense of being able to plan for or imagine what could lie ahead, but also any sense of belonging: it was only after the 1994 elections that my body felt at home

Karel Nel, *Taung*, computer-generated drawing, 1985. Produced for the poster commissioned by Phillip Tobias for the Taung Diamond Jubilee International Symposium, courtesy Karel Nel and Phillip Tobias.

enough in the country of my birth to conceive a child. Similarly, Karel, recalling the sight of the vapours rising from the trembling earth, said that what had shattered for him was the certainty about place. The earth had moved that day, and it had triggered a deep lack of settlement about permanence, about being sure of one's place.

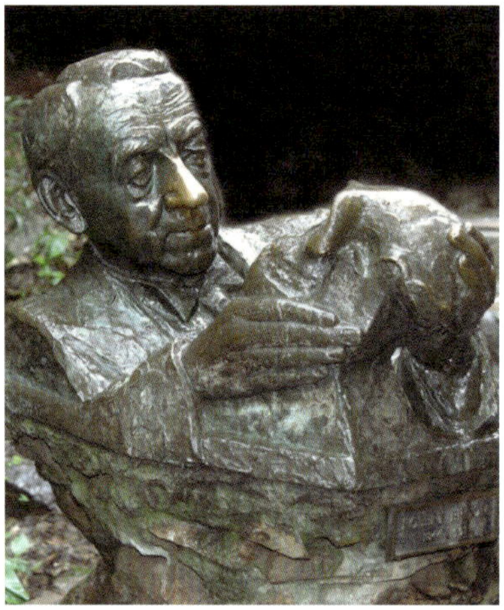

Elsa Dziomba's bronze sculpture of Robert Broom with his reconstruction of *Australopithecus Africanus* based on his discovery of a brain cast and cranial pieces found in 1936, Sterkfontein caves. Photograph taken by Karel Nel, 2005.

Time and place are potent themes in Karel's work, but the scales for both range from the relatively local and historical through the global and geological to the expanses of stellar space-time, reaching back two-thirds of the way to the Big Bang. The four works on the *Life of bone* are meditations in multiple dimensions. Karel's ability to grasp – and to forge – imaginative connections and to re-present them has developed from a capacity to absorb diverse influences from his environment.

In Rivonia, not far from us, the sculptor, Elsa Dziomba, lived. What the reason was for our first visit to her home is lost now, but it was there, among her own spare, lyrical works, books and gentle lighting, that the first actual *ushabti* either of us had ever seen was held and handled, a small ceramic figurine from a pharaoh's tomb, symbolic labour for a life beyond death. So too, at Elsa's, Karel and I gazed on the sombre visage of Mrs Ples, for Dziomba had made a cast of the Australopithicine skull.

It would have been during those childhood years too that, on a weekend outing, we would have gone down into the Sterkfontein caves. We'd looked at Dziomba's bronze of Robert Broom, his sharp nose shiny from being touched – and the skull, recognising it from the visit to the studio. Then the descent into the pitch blackness of the caves, the slightly fusty dankness, the slipperiness underfoot, the unexpected narrowings and the sudden galleries of stalactites and stalagmites glimmering in the feeble light, and then in the midst of all this strangeness, the seemingly impossible resting place for a very early ancestor of the human line … Lynne Slonimsky's poem, *The Bone Joiner*, written for Joni Brenner, brought back so vividly the strange terror that lingered long after we emerged into the Highveld sunlight: Slo writes about how she 'cried and cried for her two million years of solitude/So scared in the dark with only the drip drop of lime to keep her company'. How ever did Mrs Ples get there, so far down in the

Elsa Dziomba with her sculpture *Woman*. Collection: Johannesburg Art Gallery. Photograph taken by H.R. Klein, 1969, courtesy Esmé Berman archive.

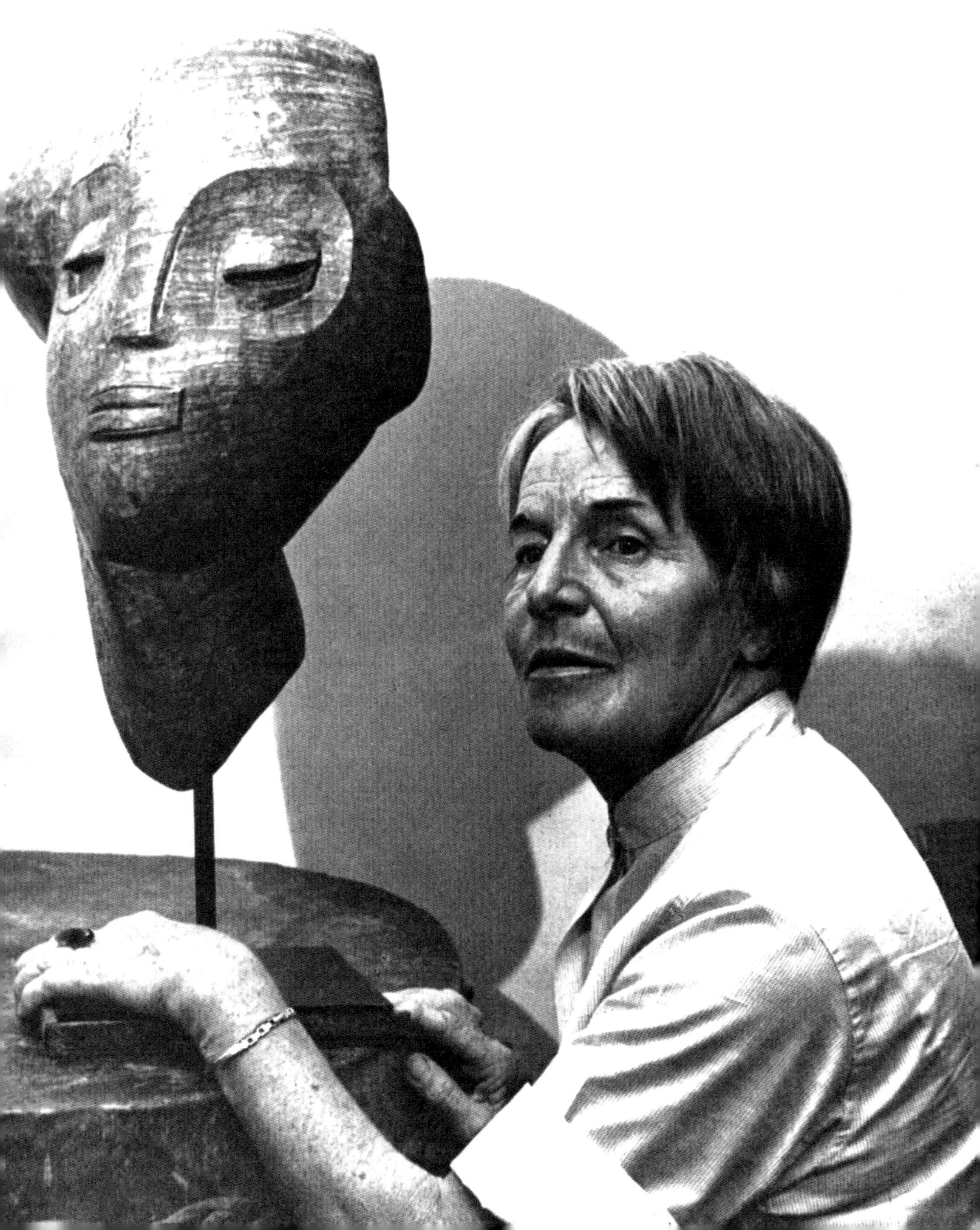

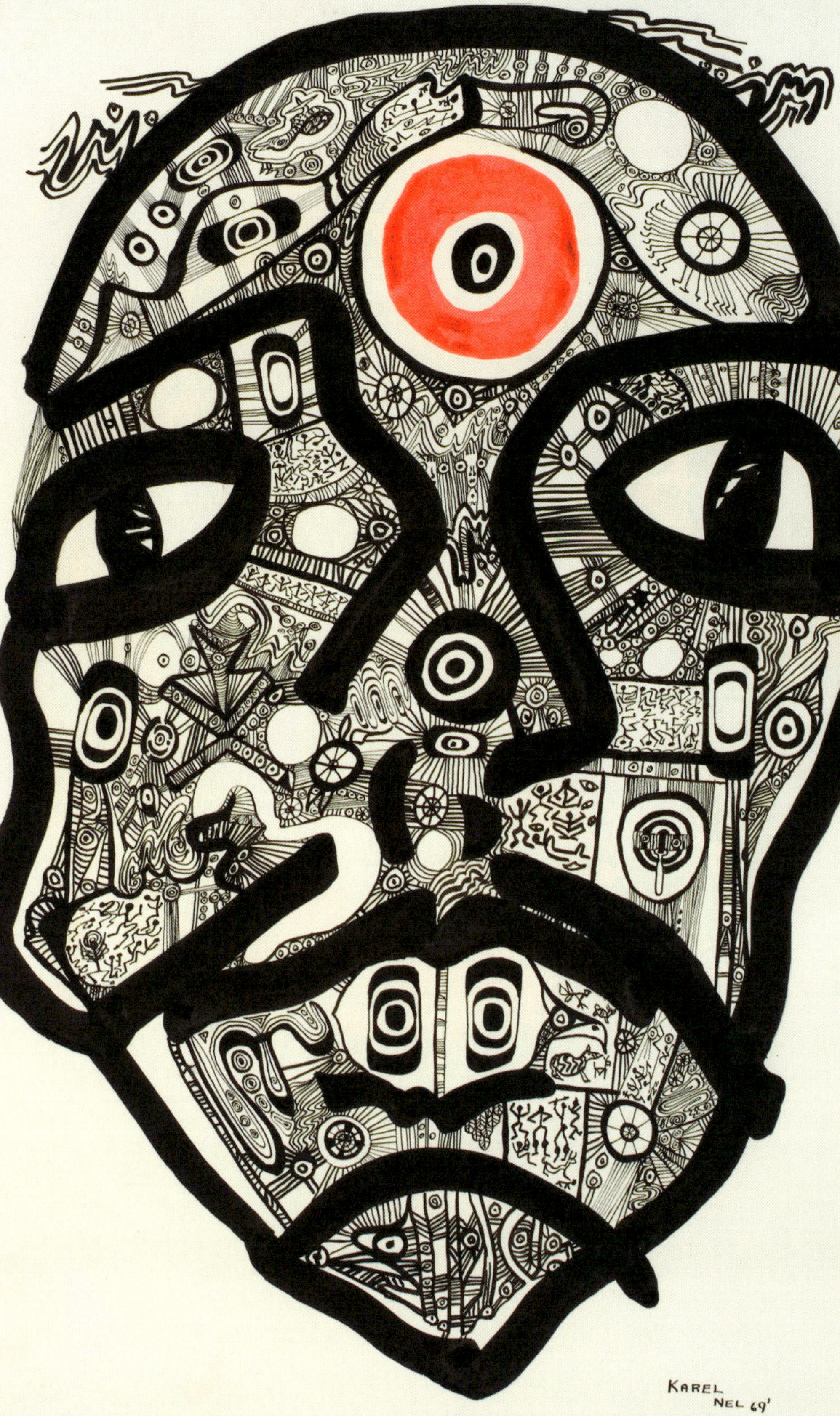
KAREL
NEL 69'

earth that she was turned to stone herself? And how, in all that winding labyrinth, was it possible that anyone would have found her all these millennia later? Although Mrs Ples seemed badly made, clumsily put together by later standards, we recognised ourselves in her and wept, like Slo did, for her untimely death, and in the safety of the car, Mom dispensed comfort along with tissues and an apple.

A large pencil drawing of a lemur skull resulted from an encounter between Karel and Walter Battiss. Karel's beloved great-uncle Pix had set up the meeting between his friend and his niece's young son, then still a schoolboy of fourteen or fifteen. At the time, Karel had been creating images using brush and ink, mostly black with some yellow or magenta. The 'bones' or primary structure of the drawing were done with a thick brush, and then the 'connective tissue' was a myriad of small details, little paintings and cross-hatchings within the larger drawing. While Karel dipped his brush and drew, his importunate sister would sit close by, and want to know how the detail emerging connected with the big picture, and Karel would have to find the words to explain himself. In retrospect, those black ink drawings drew on Miro, Picasso and more immediately on the work of Cecil Skotnes and perhaps even Battiss himself. During that seminal meeting, having looked through the works, Battiss encouraged Karel to practise realistic drawing as well, and that is what he did. But, even then, Karel's drawings were already representing inner realities, what goes on within, rather than the surfaces of things. Having satisfied himself that he could do it, Karel went on to be inventive in all sorts of mediums: with Dad's help, he created a miniature mummy with its decorated sarcophagus, and constructed a medieval monastery from balsa wood as projects for history. In between, he was carving totem poles from jarrawood sleepers, making small soapstone carvings and producing heads and pots from clay.

And all the time, he was looking: he looked at how Judith Mason drew, and then, drew differently. He appreciated the delicate tracery of her line, but made much bolder marks when he put pencil to paper. He looked at Alexis Preller's sophisticated palette and refinement of line, and considered the fact that Preller was drawing his inspiration from the Ndebele. He looked at Walter Battiss, his bright, brash colour, his playfulness, the way his interest in the rock paintings of the San was somehow reflected in his work. He looked at Irma Stern. We looked

Karel Nel, *Atman*, ink on paper, 62 x 51 cm, 1969.

together. Gallery 21 and the Goodman mostly, but the Pretoria Art Museum too – we looked together a lot, and talked and talked about what we saw. In the galleries, we saw mostly South African art including the Maggie Laubsers, Sterns, Pierneefs, Prellers and the panels and bones that Skotnes engraved, and Edoardo Villa's remarkable steel sentinels on the plaza in front of The Schlesinger Building. But we also saw the occasional Kandinsky, Picasso, Miro, Jim Dine and David Hockney. The task, and it was always in earnest, was to choose the one work we would take home if we could.

There was also Totem, where Vittorino Meneghelli displayed an everchanging trove of Yoruba *ibedjis,* the Mossi figures, the Makonde and Dan masks, the Ashanti weights, the *tijwaras* with their graceful antelope bodies and proud horns, trade beads, Senufo birds and posts, and, there was Kaplan's round the corner where I bought solid copper armbands made long ago in Angola. There too, Karel bought a Ming knife from 225 BC, the first of the currencies that would form a formidable part of his own collection. This collection serves primarily as a record of humans' ability to imbue diverse objects with value, and to incorporate them into an organic body of belief and into a living economy, but it also forms a visual lexicon and a source of metaphorical insight.

As a young boy, Karel also absorbed much from visits to Egon and Hanne Guenther's home and gallery, where he learned from Egon's collection of African objects, and the work that Egon was nurturing and promoting a group of contemporary South African artists: Skotnes, Villa, Sydney Kumalo, Ezrom Legae, Giuseppe Cattaneo and Cecily Sash. These visits were as much about talking about the genesis and values that underlay the visual manifestations as about the looking itself: the investigatory aspect was always evident in these discussions. And Karel and Dad still visit Egon and his daughter, Miriam, regularly, so that fruitful interaction lasts a lifetime.

As an adult, Karel has been a visitor of places where place itself is uncertain: he recalls experiencing the shock of having the earth shift while he studied at Berkeley, and the impact it had on him: that the earth – given of stable givens – could so rock and buck as the plates of continents ground against one another. As a family, we walked upon the sulphurous cinders of the Nea Kameni – the new

Karel Nel, *Mask*, ink on paper, 38 x 27.5 cm, 1969.

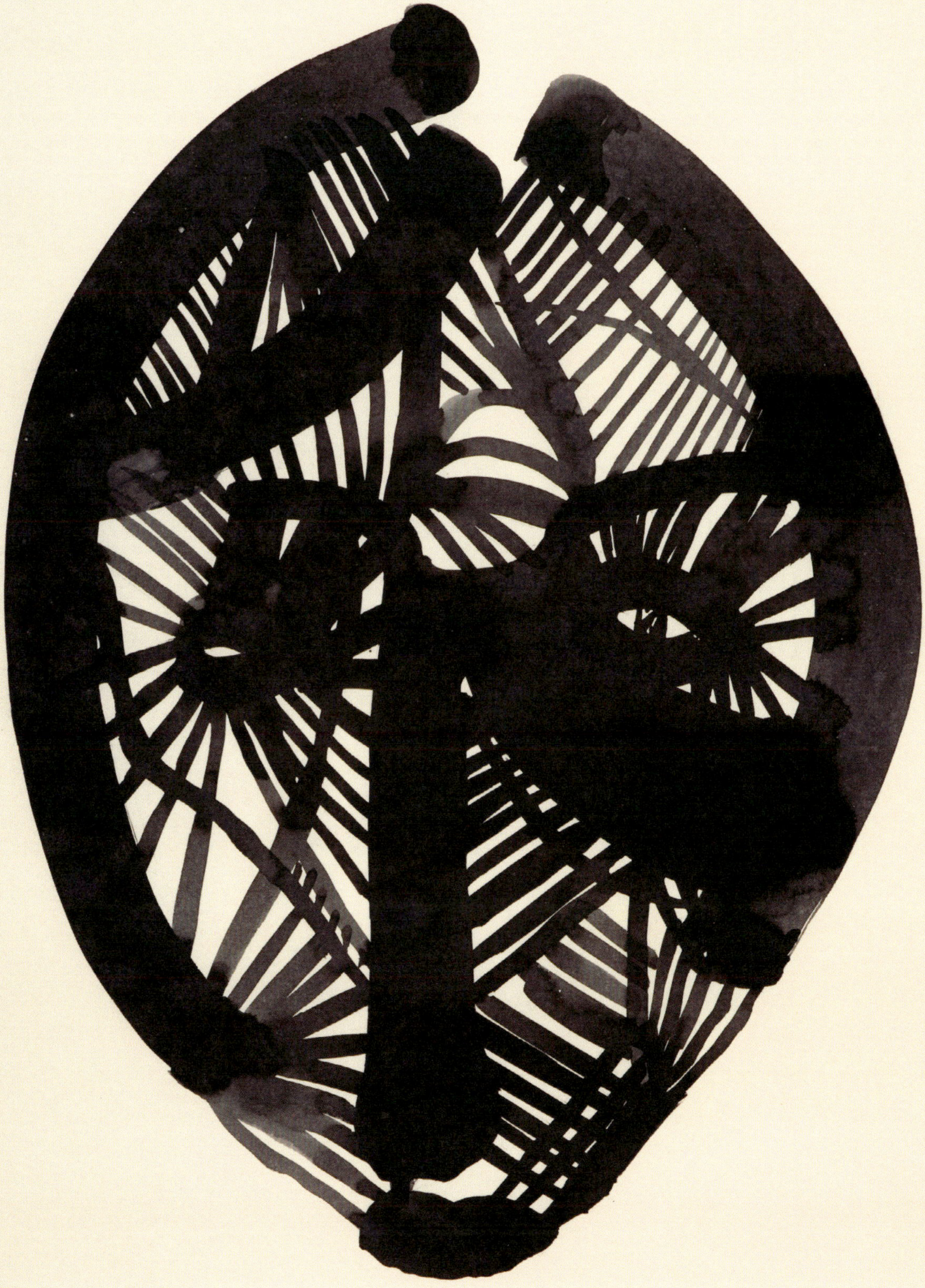
KAREL NEL. '69

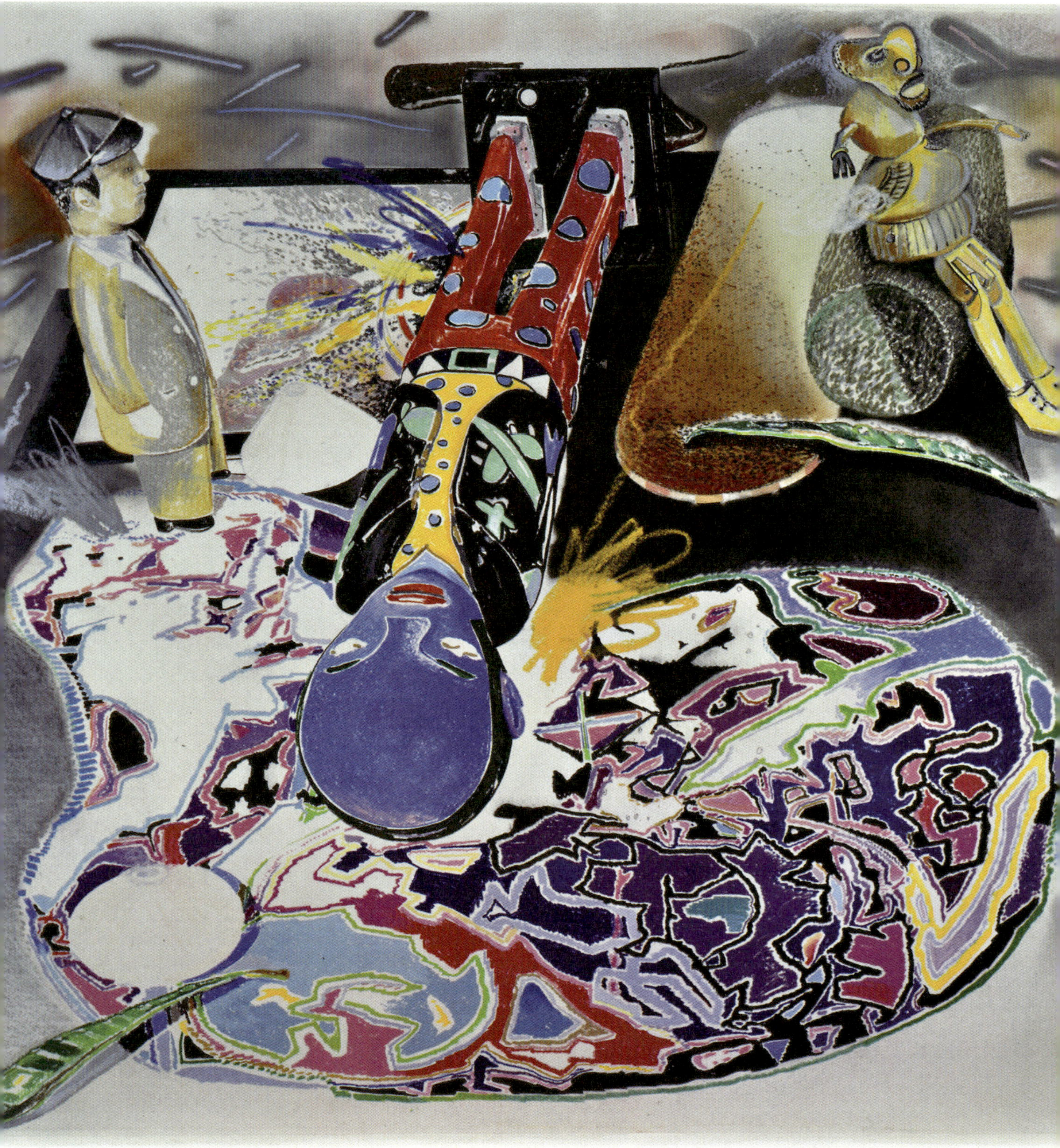

burnt ones – an islet in the caldera that is the Santorini harbour. We had gone to the Aegean island to see the archaeological remains of Thera, the early civilisation destroyed by the volcanic eruption, the origin of the myth of the destruction of Atlantis. Karel, in his annual wanderings has spent time in Hawaii where he has watched the sulphur-yellow vapours rise as the ropes of lava flow into the ocean, sputtering and setting into rock. He worked on a proposal for an environmental work on the Piton de la Fournaise on Réunion, one of the major 'hot-spot' volcanoes on the planet, which alluded both to these global pressure points of geological transformation as well as the evolutionary development of the human species. These places hold a fascination for him for a variety of reasons, but not least is the alchemical paradox of simultaneous destruction and creation. Whitesands, in the desert of New Mexico, was where humanity unleashed for the first time, energies comparable to those of a volcanic eruption. And when they found that the unprecedented release did not result in a conflagration that would obliterate the planet, they turned that misdirected creativity against Hiroshima and Nagasaki, justifying their actions as a means to end a world war. Karel gathered dust there at Whitesands, knowing that, at atomic level, this vitreous sand encapsulates Earth's consciousness of the event. At Hiroshima too, Karel gathered precious dust from the epicentre of the blast – the challenge miraculously resolved on so groomed and sensitive a site by a trench being dug for maintenance work. There too, he experienced wonderment at how the Japanese have moved beyond the horror, living vibrantly in the present. For works commemorating occasion – time and place coalesced – he has also gathered earth from Ground Zero, the site of the Bastille, and Soweto, all sites associated with shifts in human consciousness. Still, the dust, while being actual earth from the place itself, is in itself a displaced signifier: even lay people know that archaeological sites are built up layer upon layer, or that the force of rain or wind may have swept away critical clues.

The strange paradox is that, for the child whose sense of place was so deeply disturbed in the early 1960s, Rietfontein Road, Rivonia, Johannesburg – in that order – has been, and remains, consistently, continuously the place where the Nels have lived for five decades. We know no one apart from ourselves, who live

Karel Nel, *Transitional figure dreaming* pastel and pigment on bonded fibre fabric, 2m x 2m, 1987.

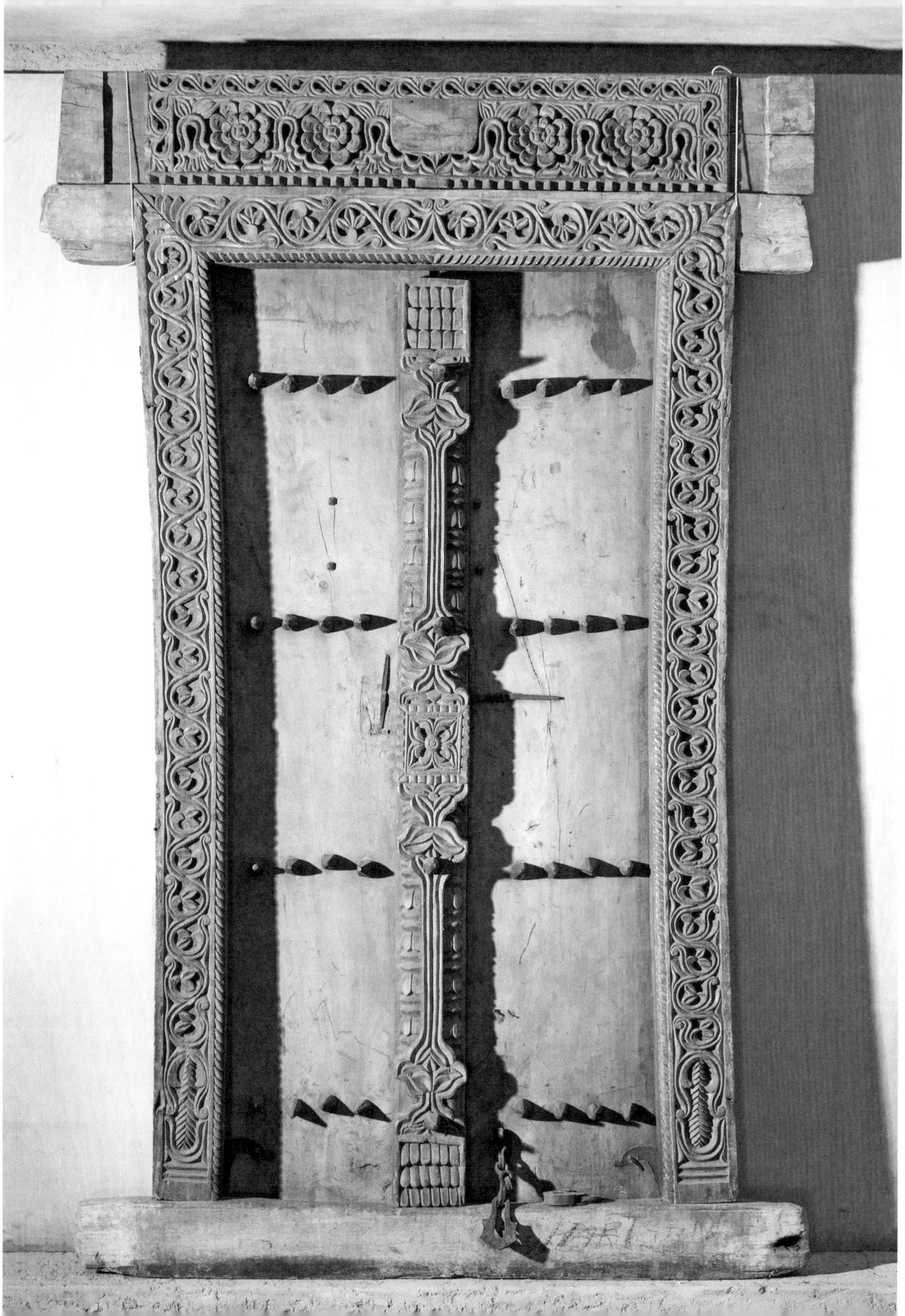

in – or have direct connection with – the home they lived in as children. This stability, this centredness, plays a critical role in identity: Karel's house, known affectionately and many-layeredly as The Mudhif stands side by side the family home. It is from here that Karel goes annually, a modern nomad, to the most cosmopolitan of destinations and the most remote of archipelagos, and it is to this studio and home that he returns.

Karel's mudhif was designed and built around a number of wooden, Zanzibari doors, four of which were collected by the Pretoria modernist architect, Norman Eaton, in the 1940s. Two of these exquisitely crafted doors were bequeathed to his long-time friend, Preller, in Eaton's will, and passed into his keeping after Eaton's untimely death. In the books that Karel and Esmé Berman, the distinguished South African art historian, wrote together on Preller, Karel concluded *Collected images* (2009) with a chapter entitled, 'The unfinished mudhif'. He writes that the construction of this building could well be regarded as Preller's last major project. Preller's mudhif was conceived as a memorial to Eaton, and an appropriate setting for the remarkable doors. The mudhif took its name and its structural inspiration from the massive reed guesthouses, built by the Marsh Arabs in southern Iraq, but the nature of the brickwork, and the stone tesserae that adorn the floor with design speak directly to Eaton's reverence for the materials used in building. Preller's own death in 1975, and that of Guna, his life partner, almost immediately afterwards, meant that the mudhif was never completed and the doors passed out of knowledge for many years, but not out of memory. The whereabouts of the Preller doors became a quest for Karel, and then suddenly, in 1984, the pair of them came up for auction and Karel, with much inner excitement, bought them. Within eighteen months, the four doors were with Karel, and the plans for his mudhif were under way. And so it is that Karel's studio and home, besides being many other wonderful things, is also an intimate connection with the lives of both Preller and Eaton. And while Karel's home does not allude as directly to the elegant parabolic arches of the Iraqi mudhifs as Preller's beautiful structure does, it nevertheless retains the airy spaciousness of the original architecture, the curved vault of the ceiling and the purpose of honouring those who visit there.

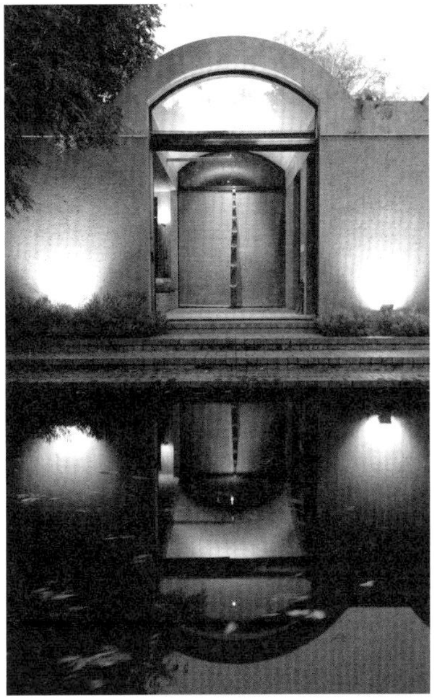

LEFT: Zanzibari door in Karel Nel's home in Rivonia, originally left to Alexis Preller in Norman Eaton's will in 1966. Photograph by John Hodgkiss, 2009.

ABOVE: View of Karel Nel's studio/home 'Mudhif', Rivonia. Photograph by John Hodgkiss, 2010.

On the wall facing his bed, Karel has Preller's 1971 painting called *You will never know*. Karel and I first stood before it in 1972 at Preller's retrospective in the beautiful modernist gallery designed by Tony Doherty, who also owned this work. At that point, Karel was still at school and I in my second year at university: we both look back to that evening as one of the high points of our lives. To be able to view a careful selection of a man's life's work, which reflected both his outer and inner journeys, was to be able to see and intuit the trajectory of Preller's life and thought. Having viewed it daily for many years, Karel has written this about it:

> Preller's rendition of the skull enables us simultaneously to see the outer details as well as to be aware of the smooth, clearly defined inner volume of space, which he often associated with the architecture of consciousness. Within the cavity, complex thought is mysteriously undertaken. For each of us, the grasp of self and the universe occurs in this small, sealed chamber … The pivotal question posed here for all is focused on the nature of both life and death, casting the sealed space as womb and tomb.[1]

Karel has mused about the title that Preller gave this work, has wondered whether it is not, at least in one sense, his answer to the question Gauguin posed when he named his 1896 existential work, *Where do we come from? What are we? Where are we going?*

Karel and I have talked and thought a lot about the fact that 'civilisation' has traditionally been associated with the advent of a settled existence, but, because of his interest in the beauty and power of the small, intimate objects associated with the pastoral societies of southern and eastern Africa, we have considered and appreciated the aesthetic refinement and complex numinous associations with portable objects such as snuff containers and snuff combs, the fertility figures ranging from the ethereal whisk-like Swazi switches to the beaded conical figures of the Ndebele, and the refined grass circlets of the Ntwanas with their ochred hair, and a beaded decoration which looks like an infinity sign. Karel has looked, and thought and written about the staffs, the meat platters, the slender milk-pails and the headrests, which embody a minimalistic way of life, a system

Alexis Preller, *You will never know*, oil on canvas, 137.5 x 137.5 cm, 1971, courtesy Karel Nel and gordonschachatcollection.

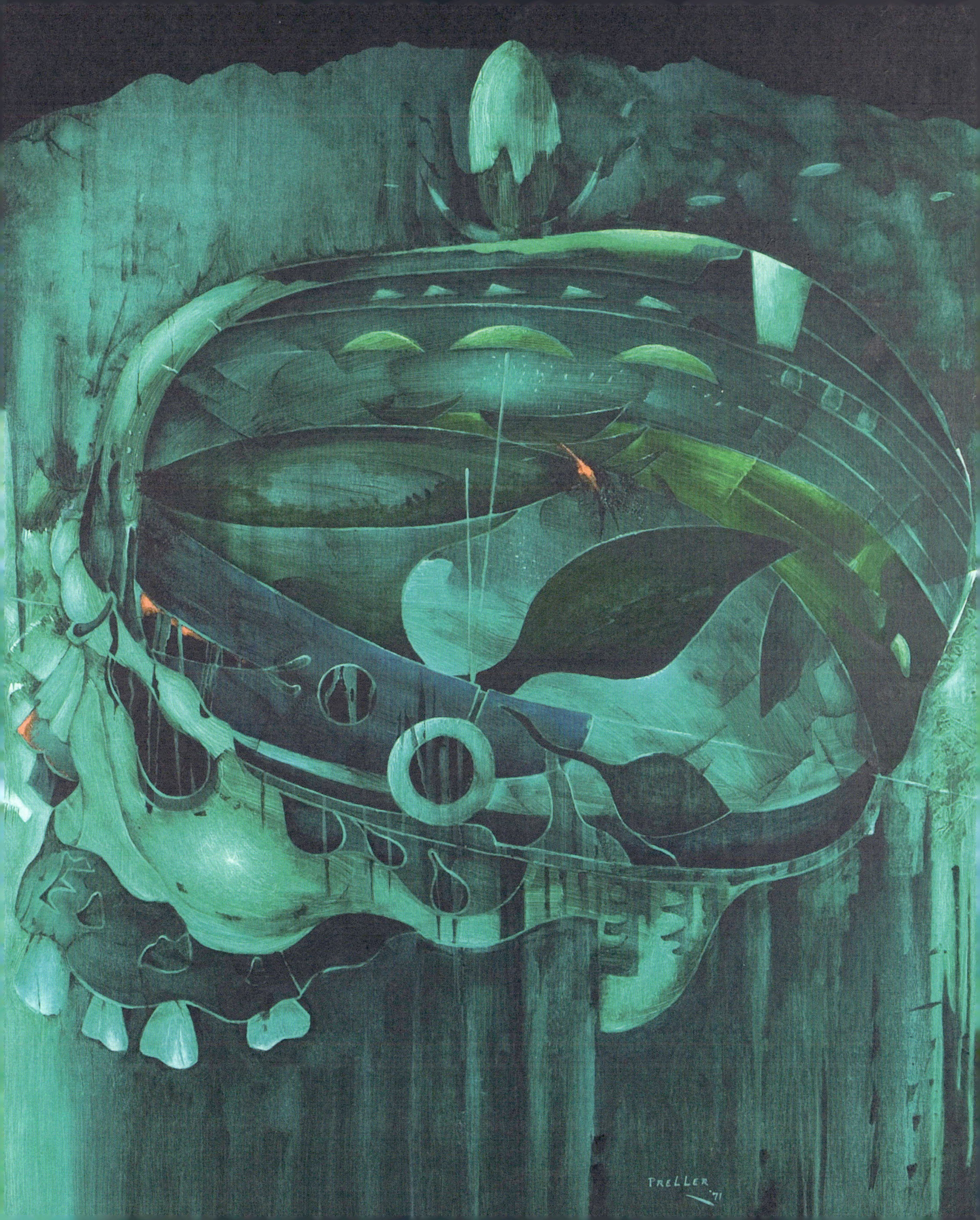
PRELLER '71

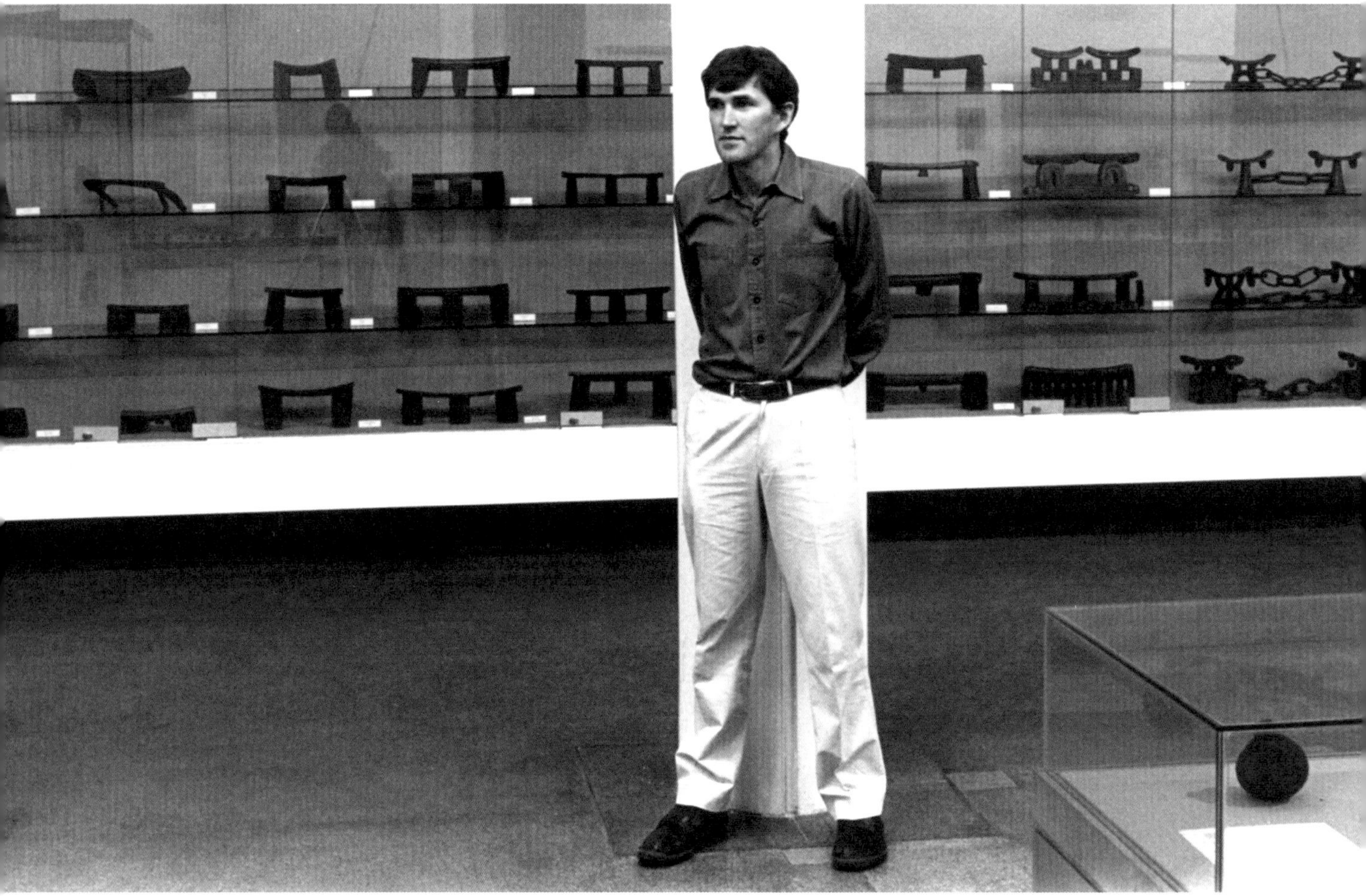

Karel Nel in front of his installation of the Brenthurst Collection headrests at the Johannesburg Art Gallery for the exhibition, *Art and Ambiguity*, 1991. Photograph taken by Bob Cnoops, 1991.

of belief and a refined sensibility. His empathy for these objects stems from, as he says, knowing and appreciating Zulu beehive huts long before he saw his first cathedral.

In 1991, the *Art and ambiguity* exhibition at the Johannesburg Art Gallery showed, for the first time, 19th-century Zulu and Tsonga pieces returned from Europe. Karel installed the headrests as a single massed display against a wall. The restrained beauty of these small practical objects, which linked their owners through dreams to the ancestral realm, put together in this way, was dazzling. In the *Life of bone* exhibition, Joni and Karel use a similar matrix to create a catacomb of Joni's skull works.

In late 1984, Phillip Tobias approached Karel with an unusual request – would he produce a poster? By hosting an international conference in January 1985, Tobias planned to honour the sixtieth anniversary of Raymond Dart's 1925 article describing and naming the first hominid species to be found in Africa. *Australopithecus africanus* would eventually give credence to Darwin's contention that the African apes are man's closest evolutionary relative. Based on his anatomical study of the fossilised skull of a small child, Dart's analysis would be catalytic in displacing the origin of man as a species from Europe. By identifying the anomalies in *Eoanthropus* – man from Europe – Dart's paper would eventually cause the Piltdown skull to be identified for the fake it is. The image of the Taung skull Karel created for the conference poster was undertaken with a company called Ideadata, and made use of the most contemporary computer technology of the time. The final image was like a radiant neural field. Like *Atman,* the conference poster reflects that it is the mental trajectory of human development that interests Karel: he sometimes talks about the fact that the same idea which created the central holes in the Blombos Cave beads drives the technology that reads the DVD you slip into your computer. At the conference, which, as a family we had decided to attend, Karel forged new friendships, especially with Don Johanson, who has been a loved visitor to Rivonia in the years since.

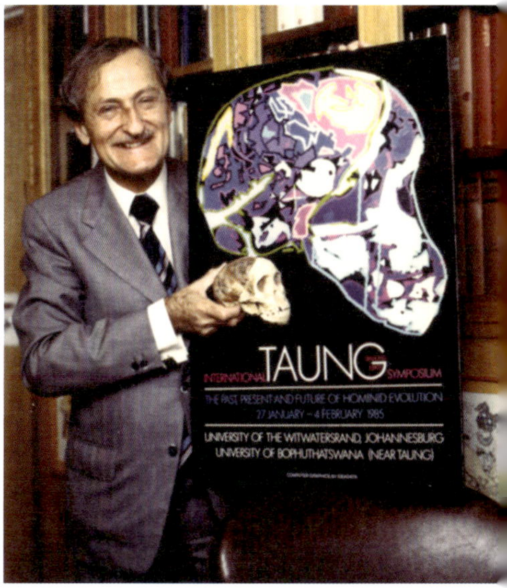
INTERNATIONAL TAUNG SYMPOSIUM
THE PAST, PRESENT AND FUTURE OF HOMINID EVOLUTION
27 JANUARY – 4 FEBRUARY 1985
UNIVERSITY OF THE WITWATERSRAND, JOHANNESBURG
UNIVERSITY OF BOPHUTHATSWANA (NEAR TAUNG)

Phillip Tobias with the poster designed by Karel Nel, courtesy Phillip Tobias, 1985.

The life of the mind, reflected in that Taung conference poster, has spun itself through Karel's work in so many different ways. Some of the early images – the whirling figures-of-eight works on the first exhibition, at the Johannesburg

Art Gallery, had their origins in meditation, and in neural patterns that quietness imprints on the screen of the mind's eye. These images were also associated with sound: just before Karel left to study in London, I found a book on Islamic calligraphy in the Rhodes library. It was one of those discoveries that literally opened both heart and mind. Poring over the book together in the weeks before he left resulted in exquisite descriptions in Karel's letters. Listening to music, conducted by the likes of Ricardo Muti and Vladimir Ashkenazy, the sinuous lines of music evoked for him mental images of the fluid strokes of the early Islamic manuscripts. The magical transformation of sound into word, the revolution of word into written mark, the power of the word to occlude what lies before and beyond the word have all been considered in Karel's work: the muezzin's cry calling the mind to focus on the ineffable; the opening of the third eye, the Ajna centre, through ancient sound practices, to the *Prelinguistic landscape* – these have been the subjects of drawings. Even the *Elegies to the forests* are visual expressions of far-reaching cries for the impact we have on the planet, and on the wisdom and knowledge of cultures other than our own.

In our parents' bedroom hangs *Sound of the rod*, one of Karel's most enigmatic works. Hovering above, or making its own space within a tracery of lines and particles, and central to the composition, is a mandorla, that internal shape defined when two circles intersect. This pure mathematical form represents the interaction of complementary opposites, the holding in balance of seemingly incompatible conceptions. In both eastern and western mystical traditions, the mandorla has come to represent the capacity to encompass the human and the divine, the inner world and the outer, life and death. It represents the threshold where the apparent contradictions of rational thought are effortlessly resolved in contemplation. The freed mind, unshackled from linear thought, moves in the realm of intuition, trusting insight, a capacity shared by both scientists and artists. When we were discussing this work again recently, Karel said the work had come to him while he was attending lectures at Berkeley by Donald Glaser, the Nobel laureate, on neural networks and perception, illustrated by the mind-teasing complexity of the dual wave-particle nature of light.

Karel Nel, *Sound of the rod*, pastel and sprayed pigment on bonded fibre fabric, 235 x 184 cm, 1989.

The idea of the threshold is also reflected in the large drawings Karel did

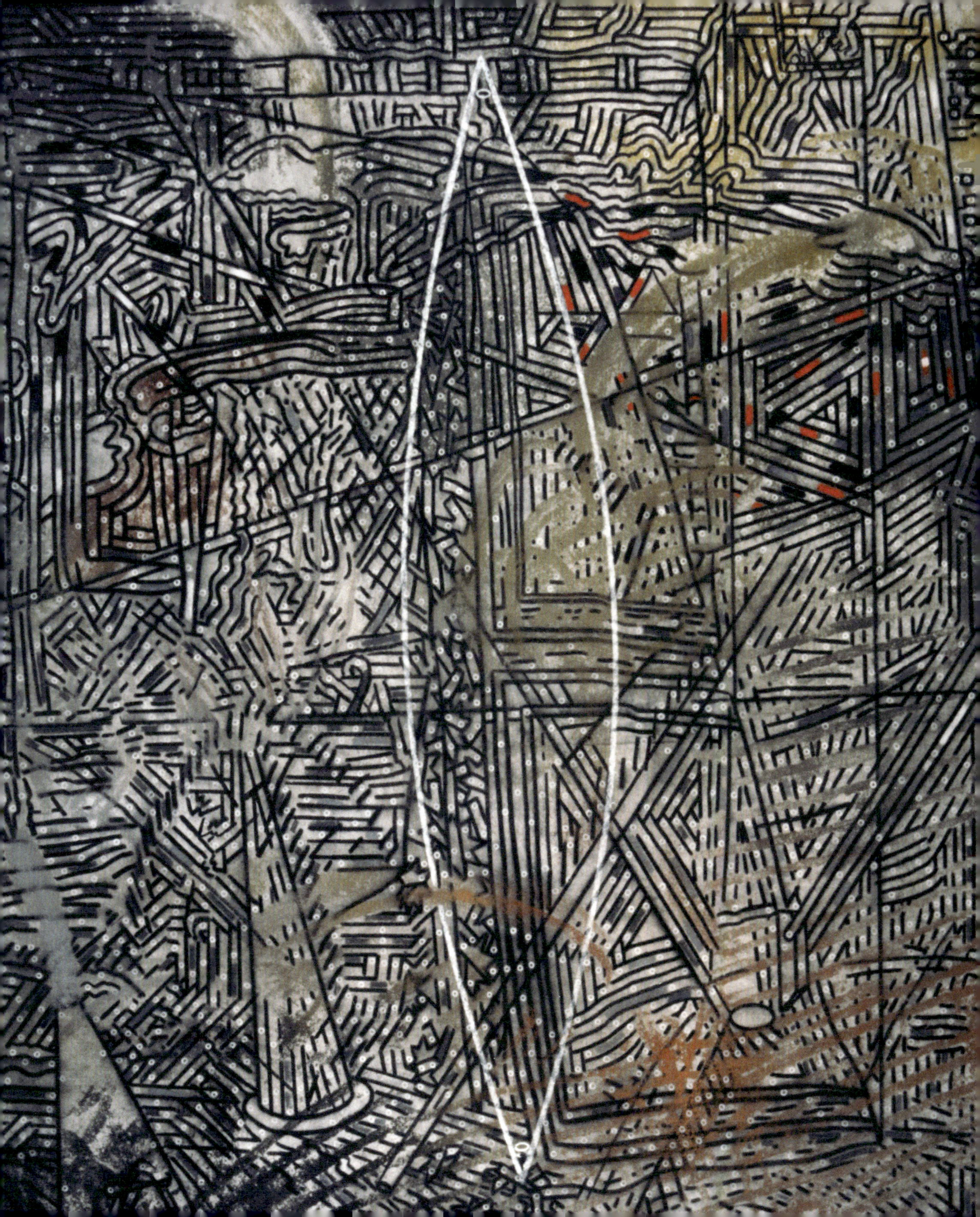

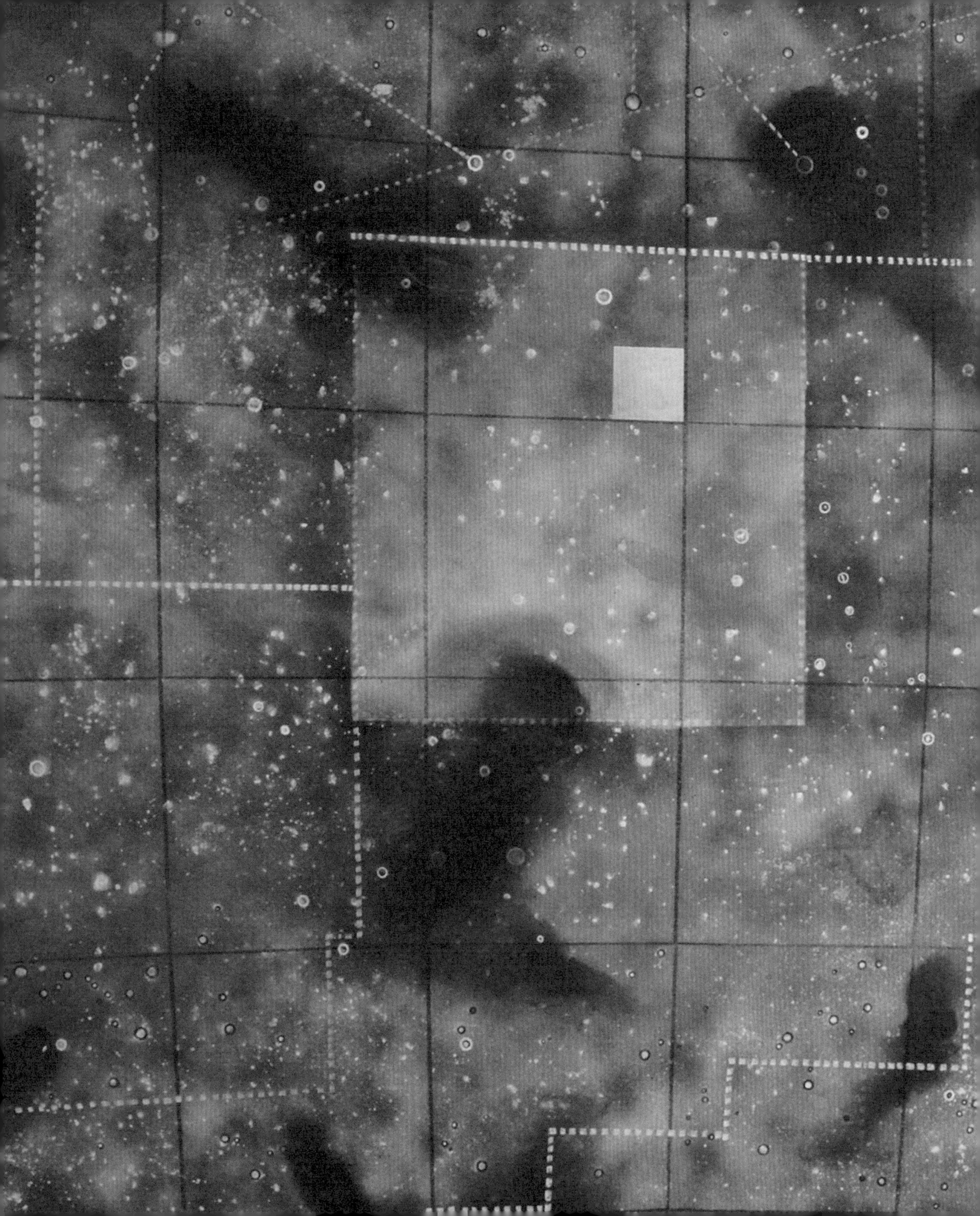

based on the rubbings of the Zanzibari doors. The doorway is the place from which it is possible to look outwards and in. Meditation is the state from which one is able to contemplate the outer reality and its inward manifestation. Karel works from the mandorla. That space allows the beginning of time to co-exist with the present – images of primaeval galaxies racing across the eye of the Hubble telescope at the speed of light on their way into the future, caught in the near present; unimaginably vast tracts of space captured on a scale that allows human perception; time and space folded and compacted, both impossibly abstract and completely real, are captured in sea salt and glittering particles of carboniferous dust, Gaia's primordial compounds.

Karel's work emanates from his remaining active within the mandorla: the sound of the rod is, after all, silence. Within that silence, bounded by the circumference of his skull, he charts the evolution of species and maps the diaspora of the cosmos, and in doing so, transforms consciousness itself. The trance maps he makes invite the reader of his work to step into that space and be transported.

Karel Nel, *Sector: two square degrees*, charcoal, pastel, specularite and sprayed pigment on bonded fibre fabric, 193 x 193 cm, 2007.

Notes

1 Berman, E and Nel, K. 2009. *Alexis Preller: Collected Images*. Johannesburg: Shelf publishing. p. 255.

Chapter 9

Conclusion

Joni Brenner and Elizabeth Burroughs

> 'Blood on ice is not a sign of death but an affirmation of life.'[1]

The work on this project, which has extended over a period of years, but which has been most intensive in the months leading up to the production of the book and the exhibition, has resulted in much that was expected, but also some surprises. One of the realisations emerging from the project has been this powerful understanding of the dual existence of life and death in the presence of bone. Far from being horrific or ghoulish, skulls, as Joni Brenner has observed, are a reminder of the power of life, of the very fact that one is alive. The work of observing and creating an image of a skull forms a bond that is specific, and that contains some element akin to knowledge of the person as well as affection for that skeletal remnant. Contemplation of the mortal remains of an unknown person focuses the attention on both the value and inevitable tenuousness of life. To live fully, one must face the knowledge of one's death.

This experience of working with skulls, far from being the grim reminder of mortality, rather blurs the lines between death and life. Joni's skulls are the embodiment of an idea, simultaneously representative of the past and the present. They talk of the cyclical transitions from life to death and back to life. Their frequent redness recalls the red ochres used in many traditional African rituals to symbolise transitions such as those of birth and death.

Joni Brenner, from *Wall of skulls*, watercolour on paper, (detail) 12.5 x 18 cm, 2010.

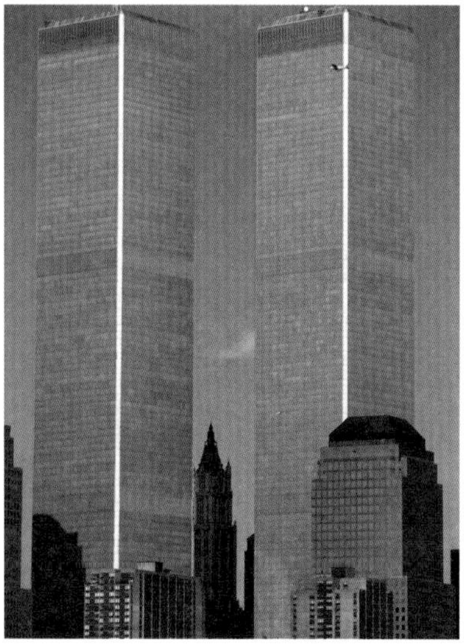

World Trade Centre Towers, New York City. Photograph courtesy Photos.com/Getty images.

While it was expected that the talking and thinking in the project would attempt to make some sense, through the bones, of the past (both very distant and the more recent past), the issue of the future of humanity loomed unexpectedly large. Our observations homed in on the fact that the conscious interment of the dead is connected to a sense of the past, and of the future – where we have come from and what will certainly be.

Bones are not, as we have been conditioned to believe, simply dour reminders of the inevitability of death. Bones are repositories of the life that was, evidence of life, even if that life is no longer. Indeed, bones have the potential to draw to themselves all manner of meaning – we can connect with them as immediate kin, regard them as evidence of the death of our foes, as the remnants of the violations of a genocide, as the continued presence of our ancestors, or part of an evolutionary puzzle. These meanings are multiple: personal, political, social, spiritual and scientific.

There is, nonetheless, something unsettling about the presence of bones. In planning the exhibition, we had thought to include a modern human skull alongside the Taung child skull and that of the chimpanzee. We soon found that on account of the Human Tissues Act, it would not be possible to publicly display human remains. The use of the Border Cave 1 skull was an acceptable alternative because, as with the Taung skull, the bone has fossilised. There was, however, not a moment's demur about putting the chimpanzee skull on display. Even before Don Johanson's essay was submitted, the oddity of what was acceptable for display, and what not, was matter for lively discussion. It seems that the stronger the possibility of identification, the stronger the taboos about what can or can't be done with bones. In a sense, the Sarah Bartmann political processes were very much about changing perceptions of her as 'other' to her as being 'the same as us'. Looking back, we consider the treatment of her remains entirely inappropriate. Different sensibilities at that time may have made her post-mortem dissection seem like a rare opportunity for science to know more. A profound fault-line runs between the human desire for knowledge and our need to respect the integrity of the one who was. Our current practices – such as displaying the chimpanzee skull when these animals, so close to us genetically, are on the verge of extinction – may, to future generations, seem just as crass as Georges Cuvier's treatment seems to us now.

Karel Nel's works for this project challenge us to identify ourselves with the dusts he has gathered from places with strong emotive associations – earth from the place early hominids first tamed fire, vitreous remains from the first atomic blast. The dust collected from sites such as Ground Zero, the Bastille, Soweto, while devoid of any obvious human remains, nonetheless carry evidentiary traces of loss and death at those places, even if they have been reduced to the merest specks of matter. As Mary Douglas argues, 'In its last phase then, dirt shows itself as an apt symbol of creative formlessness, but it is from its first phase that it derives its force.'[2] The dust from the sites that Nel has chosen for these conceptual works, while visually without obvious recognisable referents, continues to embody the affective force which derives from the original trauma. These works, therefore, have the potential to ignite strong reactions: the works are cool, dispassionate in presentation, but the matters they foreground are anything but. These works with their covert allusions to loss and death have earlier been described as abstract memento mori, and while their visual presence may be less disruptive than, say, the anamorphic skull in Holbein's *The ambassadors* of 1533, once considered, they provoke an intense, visceral response.

There is a similar paradox, or simultaneous rendering of disintegration and presence, in Gerhard Marx's work that runs through the reflections in this book: Marx uses the remains thrown away by gardeners and urban landscapers – the remnants of someone else's efforts to control, shape and tame nature. He takes these, and transforms them, preserving them in tightly controlled drawings and sculptures

Karel Nel, *Eleven*, violet pigment, earth/dust from Ground Zero, on bonded fibre fabric, 230 x 115 cm, 2001–2.

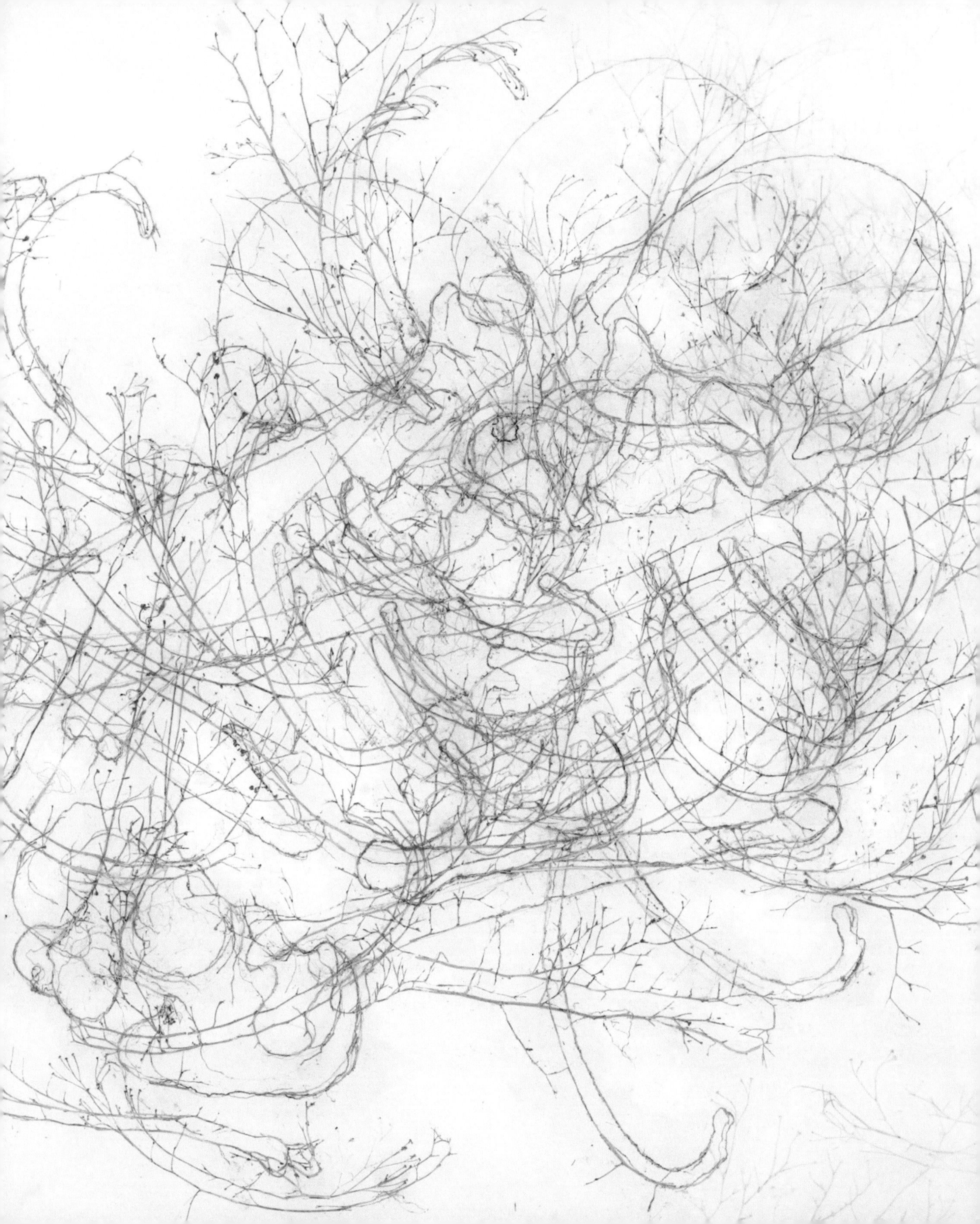

that have permanence, yet speak of disintegration and fragmented remains.

The skeletal elements delicately represented in his drawings, suggestive of the random remains of multiple bodies, prompt a taphonomic, forensic impulse to piece together a history of the fragments in order to understand the relations between parts and the significance of their original context: in short, to try and know the unknowable.

The introduction refers to Dennis Dutton's argument that art-making is an evolutionary development and that humans are driven by the desire to record experiences in the service of being able to understand themselves and the world. The forms that representations take may be visual, narrative or scientific, but all are driven by the same desire – the need to understand our place in the world.

All the conscious deliberation aside, we have chosen to end the book with Lynne Slonimsky's moving poem as it once again opens up the relationship between bones and affect.

Gerhard Marx, *Cumulus II*, plant material, acrylic paint and glue on cotton paper, 153 x 103 cm (detail), 2011.

Notes

1 Davis, W. 2009. *The Wayfinders: why ancient wisdom matters in the modern world*. Toronto: House of Anansi Press. p. 210.

2 Douglas, M. 1966. *Purity and danger*. London and New York: Routledge. p. 199.

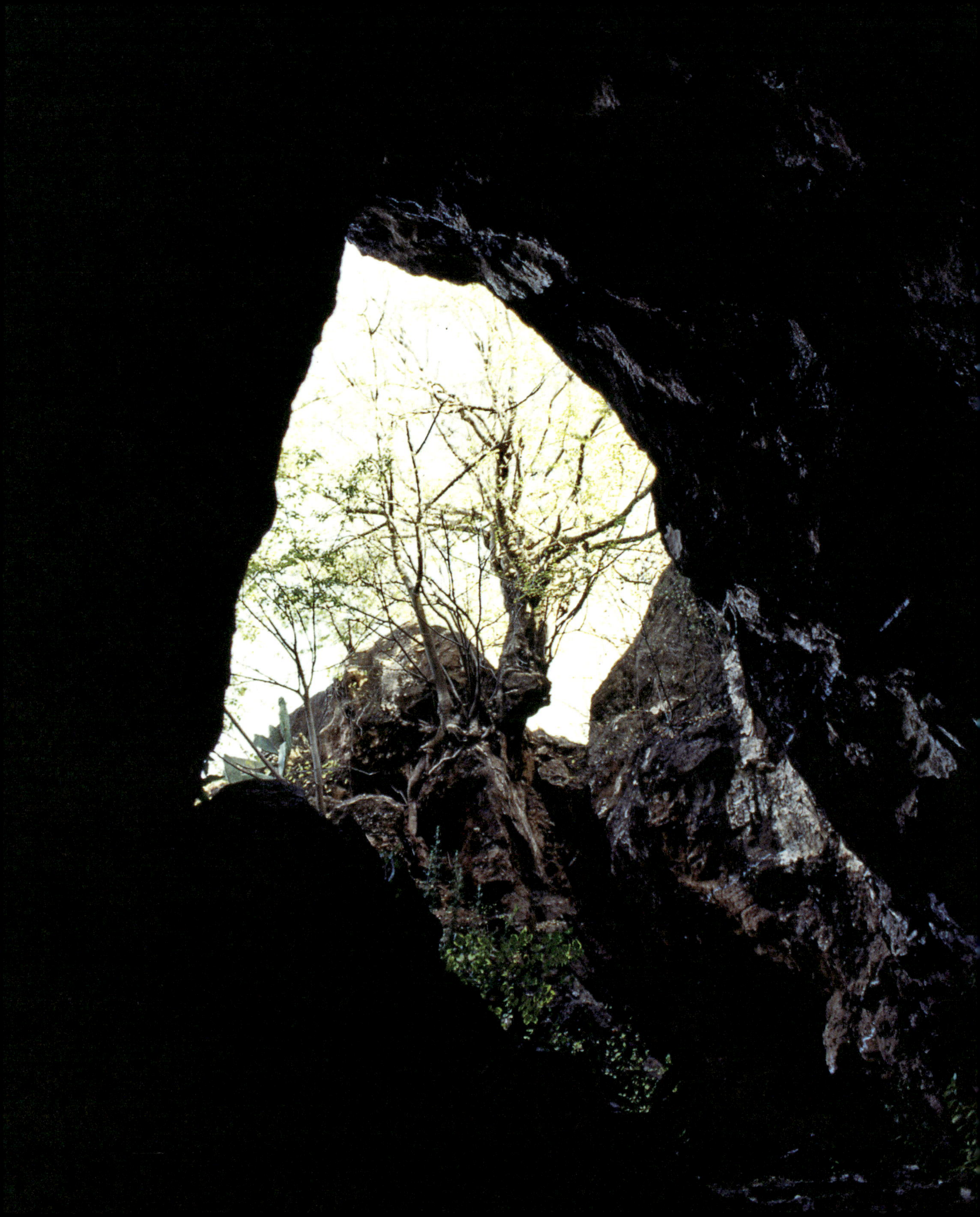

The Bone Joiner's Soul

(for Joni)

Lynne Slonimsky

When
a few days after my fifth birthday
in the close blackness of the cradle of mankind
I heard the tale of Mrs Ples
I cried and cried for her two million year solitude
so scared in the dark with only the drip drop of lime to keep her company

Half a life later, in that same womb
four foot bones then a skull were toothpicked free from their four million year tomb
Hypotheses of Little Foot's demise called up panic of
toes trying to leap or scramble from that falling earth pit
then squirming under the beast that fell down after him
When did he know he could do no more and what did he think while he waited

Humanity's story cannot be told from relics of digs and tells
DNA frozen in stone can clone beings not lives
No thing can speak history or hers
The grammar of your emotions joins flesh and blood to bones

Sterkfontein cave, Cradle of Humankind, Johannesburg. Photograph taken by Karel Nel, 1995.

Index

Please note: Page numbers in *italics* refer to photographs and images.